TEEN SUICIDE RISK

The Guilford Child and Adolescent Practitioner Series

Editors: John Piacentini, PhD, *and* John T. Walkup, MD

This series offers effective, innovative intervention strategies for today's child and adolescent practitioners. Focusing on persistent clinical challenges that cut across diagnoses and often come up in practice, books in the series present evidence-based tools for conceptualizing and addressing clients' individualized needs. These concise volumes provide what is missing from many evaluation and treatment manuals: the nuts-and-bolts techniques required for everyday clinical work. Each accessible guidebook includes a treasure trove of suggested interventions, complete with case examples, practical tips, sample dialogues, and practitioner-friendly resources, such as reproducible handouts and forms.

TEEN SUICIDE RISK

A Practitioner Guide to Screening,
Assessment, and Management

CHERYL A. KING
CYNTHIA EWELL FOSTER
KELLY M. ROGALSKI

THE GUILFORD PRESS
New York   London

© 2013 The Guilford Press
A Division of Guilford Publications, Inc.
72 Spring Street, New York, NY 10012
www.guilford.com

Printed in the United States of America

This book is printed on acid-free paper.

Last digit is print number: 9   8   7   6   5   4   3   2   1

The authors have checked with sources believed to be reliable in their efforts to provide
information that is complete and generally in accord with the standards of practice that
are accepted at the time of publication. However, in view of the possibility of human
error or changes in behavioral, mental health, or medical sciences, neither the authors,
nor the editor and publisher, nor any other party who has been involved in the preparation or publication of this work warrants that the information contained herein is in every
respect accurate or complete, and they are not responsible for any errors or omissions or
the results obtained from the use of such information. Readers are encouraged to confirm
the information contained in this book with other sources.

Library of Congress Cataloging-in-Publication Data

King, Cheryl A. Polewach, 1955–
    Teen suicide risk : a practitioner guide to screening, assessment, and management /
by Cheryl A. King, Cynthia Ewell Foster, and Kelly M. Rogalski.
        pages cm. — (The Guilford child and adolescent practitioner series)
        Includes bibliographical references and index.
        ISBN 978-1-4625-1019-1 (hard cover : alk. paper)
        1. Teenagers—Suicidal behavior.   2. Suicidal behavior—Risk factors. 3. Teenagers—
Mental health.   4. Suicide—Prevention.   I. Ewell Foster, Cynthia.   II. Rogalski,
Kelly M.   III. Title.
        RJ506.S9K56 2013
        616.85′844500835—dc23
                                                                            2013004793

About the Authors

Cheryl A. King, PhD, ABPP, is Professor in the Departments of Psychiatry and Psychology at the University of Michigan, where she serves as Director of the Youth Depression and Suicide Prevention Research Program and the Institute for Human Adjustment. She is board certified as a clinical child and adolescent psychologist. Dr. King has a longstanding record as a clinical educator and public policy advocate, and has conducted workshops across the United States and abroad on clinical practice with suicidal children, adolescents, and young adults. She has also written widely on topics related to youth suicide prevention, including research that has informed best practices in suicide risk recognition, assessment, and intervention with adolescents and young adults. Dr. King is a Fellow of the American Psychological Association and Past President of the Society for Clinical Child and Adolescent Psychology, the Association of Psychologists in Academic Health Centers, and the American Association of Suicidology.

Cynthia Ewell Foster, PhD, is Clinical Assistant Professor in the Department of Psychiatry at the University of Michigan and Director of the University Center for the Child and Family. Dr. Ewell Foster has significant training and experience in providing evidence-based interventions for youth struggling with depression and suicide risk. She serves as a clinical educator for new mental health professionals in psychiatry, psychology, and social work. Her research interests involve community- and school-based interventions for youth at risk for depression and suicide.

Dr. Ewell Foster has recently served as the Evaluation Consultant to the State of Michigan's Garrett Lee Smith Suicide Prevention Grant.

Kelly M. Rogalski, MD, is a pediatric psychiatrist and Medical Director of Outpatient Pediatric Psychiatry at Henry Ford Health System in southeastern Michigan, which is a 2011 Malcolm Baldridge National Quality Award winner for performance excellence and innovation, notably for its work in improving depression care to reduce suicide. Her research interests include quality improvement work in behavioral health. Dr. Rogalski is also a voluntary faculty member at Wayne State University School of Medicine, where she is involved in teaching medical students, residents, and nurse practitioner students.

Acknowledgments

This book is the culmination of many years of clinical practice and consultation, teaching, and applied research related to screening, assessing, and managing the care of teens at elevated risk for suicide. We have had many influential teachers along the way, including our students, who have "kept us on our toes," challenged us to respond to tough questions and help them with difficult cases, and shared with us their fresh ideas and clinical successes. We also owe a debt of gratitude to the many clinical scientists who conducted the rigorous and often painstaking research that informs practice with these teens and is included within this book. Finally, we thank our patients and clients—the at-risk teens and their families—who have been some of our most memorable teachers. As readers are undoubtedly aware, clinical science often falls short when we ask, "Exactly what is this teen's level of risk?" or "What is the best step to take next for this individual teen, given these family values and the services available in this community?" And even when we do have pertinent scientific evidence, no one disputes the importance of considering the unique backgrounds, values, and preferences of different teens and families. These teens and their families continue to teach us about emotional pain, hope, and the importance of compassion.

Rather than offer prescriptive guidelines, we chose to write an evidence-informed practitioner guidebook that points to the scientific evidence while also emphasizing compassionate care, the integration of new scientific findings over time, and consultation with other professionals. In keeping with this emphasis on consultation, we wish to acknowledge the extraordinarily helpful input we have received from many of our thoughtful colleagues in the field. In particular, we would like to thank Joan Asarnow, Lanny Berman, Rebecca Fatzinger, Julie Goldstein-Grumet, David Goldston, Gregory Hanna, David Jobes, Anne Kramer, David Litts, Nicole Nugent, and David Rudd. Each of these individuals reviewed one or more of the chapters and appendices and provided helpful, constructive suggestions for improvement. We would also like to acknowledge the child and adolescent psychiatry fellows in the Department of Psychiatry at the University of Michigan who reviewed the content and provided valuable input during their writers' workshop, with a special emphasis on how we could make the information most accessible to clinicians. Finally, completion of this book would not have been possible without the help of our highly skilled and thoughtful research assistants, Ryan Hill, Adam Horwitz, and Kiel Opperman, who assisted with literature reviews, preparing references, the creation of tables and figures, and editing.

There are many others who have made critically important contributions to our thinking and the content of this book, and who have provided support, guidance, and inspiration to each of us. Dr. King thanks Dr. Cynthia Pfeffer and Dr. David Brent, who each served as a role model and research advisor to her at a critical point during her career, and her generous and supportive colleagues and friends in the American Association of Suicidology and the American Foundation for Suicide Prevention. She also thanks the survivors of suicide who bear witness to its tragedy and continue to advocate passionately for continued research and improved clinical practice. Dr. Ewell Foster would like to thank Dr. Judy Garber, her first academic mentor, who instilled a desire to understand and, by extension, to help young people at risk for depression and suicide, and Dr. Joseph Durlak, who inspired a passion for community advocacy and public health approaches to prevention and intervention. In addition, Dr. Ewell Foster would like to recognize the community of Garrett Lee Smith grantees across the nation who are working tirelessly with the support of the Substance Abuse and Mental Health Services Administration and the Suicide

Prevention Resource Center to build real and lasting capacity for youth suicide prevention. Finally, she would like to extend heartfelt thanks to Dr. Cheryl A. King, her mentor for the past 10 years. Dr. Rogalski would like to thank a dear mentor, Dr. Lisa MacLean, for advocating for her development throughout residency and beyond. In addition, she thanks Dr. Ed Coffey for promoting her ongoing growth and learning during the early years of her career.

Finally, we would like to acknowledge individuals in our personal lives who have made this book possible.

Cheryl A. King: Throughout the more than 25 years of my work in youth suicide prevention, my husband, Steve, and my daughters, Janna and Michelle, have been the foundation and joy of my life. Thank you! In the whirlwind of an academic's life—with the multitasking and deadlines that come with the roles of clinical researcher, clinician and clinical educator, and administrator—I have been fortunate to experience much calm and centeredness. I attribute this to my parents, who taught me to work hard and embrace commonsense values, and to our growing family, which embraces connectedness, personal development, and a life of many adventures.

Cynthia Ewell Foster: Enormous thank-yous to my parents, Mal and Daisy Ewell, for years and years of unconditional love and encouragement (and for that college education!), and to my husband, Chuck, and our three amazing kids, Charlie, Virginia, and Jacob. They definitely add sparkle, fun, and meaning to every day.

Kelly M. Rogalski: Thank you to my husband, Joe, for encouraging my love of learning. From the moment I began this project, he supported every step. He has been there through the long journey of medical school, residency, and fellowship; now, as I pursue my career, he continues to support what is clearly my passion and not just a job. I am blessed to have Joe balance my serious side and add fun and spontaneity to create wonderful memories.

Authors' Note

While this book focuses on screening, assessment, and management with suicidal teens, we do not intend to define the standard of care. Our hope is to provide a useful resource for working with these teens. Each case is unique and presents an individual set of clinical and risk management issues. Nothing can replace appropriate training, experience, clinical supervision, and consultation when working with this challenging population of patients.

Contents

Contents

CHAPTER ONE

Introduction

CHAPTER OBJECTIVES

▶ Describe objectives and organization of the practitioner guide.

▶ Discuss practitioner challenges inherent in work with suicidal teens.

▶ Present a classification system for suicidal and self-injurious behavior.

▶ Present a rationale for evidence-based, systematic approach to screening, risk assessment, and care management.

We are writing this practitioner guide to provide you with both a *clear and systematic strategy* and a *set of practical tools* for identifying and working effectively and safely with teens at elevated risk for suicidal behavior and suicide. If your practice includes teens, you almost certainly have worked with these at-risk teens. A concern about suicide risk—whether due to a suicide attempt, a text message or diary entry indicating suicidal intent, or an expression of suicidal thoughts—is the most common mental health emergency in this age group.

Our objectives for this practitioner guide are as follows:

- *To describe the challenge of teen suicide risk for practitioners,* how we *classify teens' self-harmful and suicidal behavior,* and the *value of a systematic and structured clinical approach.*
- To present an *up-to-date, evidence-based, and accessible overview of risk and protective factors* for teen suicidal behavior and suicide, with checklists and tools that can be used in your setting.
- To review the *basic principles of suicide risk screening* and provide clear guidelines for suicide risk screening in your setting.
- To describe the *key components of a comprehensive suicide risk assessment,* with specific strategies for how to conduct a specific inquiry about suicidal thoughts and impulses, how to make use of self-report questionnaires, and how to modify the assessment strategy for your setting.
- To provide an *evidence-based suicide risk formulation strategy* that incorporates an easy-to-use checklist, guidelines for integrating risk assessment findings, and guidelines for charting the formulation.
- To provide a *safety plan template (crisis response plan),* in addition to step-by-step instructions about how to develop such a plan with the teen.
- To present *strategies for partnering with at-risk teens and their parents,* providing psychoeducation and involving them in a collaborative risk assessment, and developing safety plans, safety monitoring, and facilitating treatment adherence.
- To *provide tools and strategies for working effectively with schools,* and for assisting parents in developing a partnership with school personnel and facilitating a collaborative care approach to helping the suicidal teen.
- To describe *how to minimize your potential for legal problems* through systematic risk formulation and care management, strong documentation, and a consideration of confidentiality versus safety concerns.

ORGANIZATION OF THIS PRACTITIONER GUIDE

We have organized this practitioner guide in a manner that allows you to access easily all of the key strategies and tools for screening, comprehensive risk assessment, risk formulation, safety planning, partnering with parents and teens, and ongoing care management. Our goal is to provide you with practical guidelines that you can turn to when needed, even if pressed for time.

Each chapter begins with a list of objectives that enable you to easily ascertain chapter topics. Then, depending on chapter content, the text is supplemented by one or more of the following: easy-to-find boxes that delineate key points, **Clinical Notes** that emphasize clinical recommendations, tables that present more detailed information, sample dialogues, and completed clinical forms. (Note: The Appendices contain blank clinical forms that are reproducible for your use.) Taken together, we provide you with *clinically relevant information* and a *wide array of clinical tools* that we believe will be helpful as you strive to diminish the suicide risk and improve the lives of at-risk teens in your practice.

THE CHALLENGES FOR PRACTITIONERS

High Prevalence of Teen Suicide Risk

Most practitioners who work with teens will encounter suicidal teens—regardless of whether they work in an outpatient clinic, psychiatric hospital, emergency setting, or school setting. Some practitioners encounter these teens on a relatively frequent basis because the prevalence rates for suicidal thoughts and attempts in this age group are strikingly high. Based on nationally representative data from the 2011 Youth Risk Behavior Survey (YRBS), 15.8% of high school students have seriously considered attempting suicide in the preceding year, and 12.8% have made a plan about how they would attempt suicide. Moreover, 7.8% of high school students report that they have attempted suicide one or more times in the preceding year and 2.4% report having made a suicide attempt that resulted in an injury, poisoning, or an overdose that had to be treated by a doctor or nurse (Centers for Disease Control and Prevention[CDC], 2012b). That is, one out of every 50 high school students in the United States seeks medical care each year due to a suicide-attempt injury.

Depending on your setting and position, your role may be to conduct a brief suicide risk screen and then refer the teen for a comprehensive suicide risk assessment, if needed. This may be the case if you work in a school setting. Alternatively, if you practice in an emergency department or mental health setting, your role may be to conduct the screen and the comprehensive risk assessment, arrive at a solid case formulation, and make recommendations for disposition and treatment. It is also possible that you are responsible for the ongoing treatment and care management of one or more suicidal teens. This book provides you with the clinical knowledge and tools needed to implement suicide risk screens; conduct comprehensive risk assessments; develop immediate intervention plans, including safety plans; and communicate effectively with teens, parents/guardians, and school personnel concerning suicide risk and risk management.

Practitioner Tensions Are Common

Clinical practice with suicidal or potentially suicidal teens is challenging. One of the most common dilemmas is the tension that may develop between the clinician's desire to establish strong rapport and take a collaborative, growth-oriented, therapeutic approach, and his or her desire to take control and manage safety concerns. These are not mutually exclusive, but they can run counter to each other. Realistic fears and anxieties related to the teen's safety and possible suicide risk, in addition to liability concerns, can result in a desire for control and perhaps an overemphasis on hospitalization as a therapeutic strategy. Without clear and systematic approaches to screening, assessing, and managing the suicidal teen, the clinician may feel he or she is all alone and working to string together a series of assessment and crisis management responses. We believe the systematic strategy described in this guide will lessen your anxiety and enable you to more easily provide high-quality care.

A second common challenge pertains to resource limitations. Our goal to provide comprehensive treatment and care management frequently runs up against limited services available in the community. It may be that the teen's family has no health insurance and a limited ability to pay out of pocket. It is also possible, however, that the community itself does not have a sufficient number of mental health professionals trained in evidence-based treatments, enough psychiatrists and pediatricians who have expertise in pediatric psychopharmacology and are willing to take on the medication management of high-risk teens, or enough space in psychiatric inpatient units. Whereas combination treatment—psychosocial and psychopharmacology treatments—may be the most effective for some suicidal teens, especially those who struggle with clinical depression, such treatment can be a costly option that is not readily available to many families. Furthermore, although such combination treatment has been associated with reduced depression severity among adolescents, we do not have evidence to suggest that it can be related directly to reductions in suicide and suicide attempt risk. It becomes even more challenging to wrap these mental health treatments into a more comprehensive package of services that includes psychoeducation for the family and community-based services to address broader parent and family needs.

This practitioner guide focuses on what you can do. The systematic, evidence-based approach that we recommend will enable you to take active, positive steps to screen adolescents; conduct well-informed risk assessments; manage the care of suicidal adolescents; and communicate effectively with parents, adolescents, and school personnel throughout the process. We provide rich background information, an up-to-date overview of clinical strategies, and practical clinical tools to enable you to approach this challenging work systematically and with confidence, consulting with others and providing stepped-up care as needed.

CLASSIFICATION AND DEFINITIONS

Self-Injurious Behavior, Suicidal Behavior, and Suicide

Several different sets of terms have been used to refer to the spectrum of suicidal ideation and behavior. This inconsistency, sometimes found even among clinical providers who work in the same setting, can compromise communication among the teen's providers. It also hampers advancements in our field.

Fortunately, the importance of having and using a uniform classification system with standardized terminology is now widely accepted. Such classification systems have been published and widely disseminated (O'Carroll, Berman, Maris, & Moscicki, 1996; Silverman, Berman, Sanddal, O'Carroll, & Joiner, 2007). Most recently, the CDC has developed a set of uniform definitions and recommended data elements on self-directed violence (Crosby, Ortega, & Melanson, 2011). These are delineated in Table 1.1.

TABLE 1.1. The CDC's Uniform Definitions of Suicide and Suicidal Behavior

Term	Definition
Self-directed violence	Behavior that is self-directed and deliberately results in injury or the potential for injury to oneself. This does not include behaviors such as gambling, substance use, or other risk-taking activities, such as excessive speeding in motor vehicles.
Nonsuicidal self-directed violence	Behavior that is self-directed and deliberately results in injury or the potential for injury to oneself. There is no evidence, whether implicit or explicit, of suicidal intent.
Suicidal self-directed violence	Behavior that is self-directed and deliberately results in injury or the potential for injury to oneself. There is evidence, whether implicit or explicit, of suicidal intent.
Undetermined self-directed violence	Behavior that is self-directed and deliberately results in injury or the potential for injury to oneself. Suicidal intent is unclear based on the available evidence.

(continued)

6

TABLE 1.1. *(continued)*

Term	Definition
Nonsuicidal self-injurious behavior	A self-inflicted, potentially harmful behavior with no intent to die as a result of the behavior, such as to affect external circumstances or internal state.
Interrupted self-directed violence—by other	A person takes steps to injure self but is stopped by another person prior to fatal injury. The interruption can occur at any point during the act, such as after the initial thought or after onset of behavior.
Interrupted self-directed violence—by self	A person takes steps to injure self but is stopped by self prior to fatal injury.
Other suicidal behavior, including preparatory acts	Acts or preparation toward making a suicide attempt, but before potential for harm has begun. This can include anything beyond a verbalization or thought, such as assembling a method (e.g., buying a gun) or preparing for one's death by suicide (e.g., writing a suicide note).
Suicide attempt	A nonfatal, self-directed, potentially injurious behavior with any intent to die as a result of the behavior. A suicide attempt may or may not result in injury.
Suicide	Death caused by self-inflicted injurious behavior with any intent to die as a result of the behavior.

According to the definitions in Table 1.1, a suicide attempt is a nonfatal self-inflicted behavior that (1) had the potential to cause injury (whether or not it did), and (2) was associated with some degree of intent to die. If we have absolutely no information from a teen about suicidal intent (and no ancillary information such as a written note or a parent reporting that the teen verbalized suicidal intent), the behavior would be undetermined (intent) self-injurious behavior. Nonsuicidal self-injurious behavior (NSSI) is the appropriate term if it is clear that the teen had no suicidal intent at all. This may be the case with *some* instances of wrist cutting (scratching) as well as with behaviors such as self-inflicted burns or the carving of initials on the teen's arm or leg. Recent data indicates that NSSI is associated with elevated risk of a suicide attempt, which is discussed further in Chapter 2.

A SYSTEMATIC RISK ASSESSMENT AND CARE MANAGEMENT APPROACH

Best Practices: An Evidence-Based Approach

In this practitioner guide we emphasize the importance of evidence-based assessment and intervention, or what is more commonly referred to as evidence-based practice. In the United States, the national professional organizations in psychology, social work, and medicine have each provided definitions of such practice. The American Psychological Association (APA) endorses the following definition: "*Evidence-based practice in psychology* (EBPP) is the integration of the best available research with clinical expertise in the context of patient characteristics, culture, and preferences" (APA, 2006). Placing a similar emphasis on the role of research, the National Association of Social Workers (NASW, 2009) provides the following definition: "Evidence-based practices are interventions shown to be effective through strong scientific research." The American Medical Association (AMA) definition expands on these definitions to address the role of the provider, offering the following definition at *www.jamaevidence. com*: "The conscientious, explicit, and judicious use of current best evidence in making decisions about the care of individual patients. Evidence-based clinical practice (or evidence-based health care) requires integration of individual clinical expertise and patient preferences with the best available external clinical evidence from systematic research, and consideration of available resources" (AMA, 2012).

In this book, we present the evidence base that is currently available to guide suicide risk assessment and care management. In some areas, such as the ideal interval between suicide risk assessments, a strong evidence base for decision making is unavailable; however, some data are available to guide the recommendations (e.g., documented increase in suicide risk following psychiatric hospitalization). We provide the available evidence, understanding that your client or patient may not exactly fit the usual research subject because of a multiplicity of factors, including co-occurring mental disorders combined with severe psychosocial trauma, or a particular cultural background or value system. In these instances, you will need to use your clinical judgment to guide you in providing the best possible care that is grounded in the current evidence base. It is also possible that you will need to make some cultural adaptations in your communication style to facilitate a working alliance with the teen and family. These adaptations and modifications can be layered onto the existing evidence base, but should not be contradictory to or inconsistent with it.

Core Competencies: A Consensus

Several professional groups have considered practice recommendations for working with suicidal adolescents or suicidal individuals in general. In addition to practice recommendations published by the American Psychiatric Association (2003) and the American Academy of Child and Adolescent Psychiatry (2001), the Substance Abuse and Mental Health Services Administration of the U.S. Department of Health and Human Services (DHHS) funded an initiative to identify the *core competencies* needed to assess and manage suicide risk. This was a response to a recommendation in the *National Strategy for Suicide Prevention* (U.S. DHHS, 2001), which noted that many training programs for mental health professionals—social workers, counselors, psychologists, psychiatrists—provide little or inadequate training in assessing and managing suicide risk. As noted in the *National Strategy for Suicide Prevention* (U.S. DHHS, p. 79), many of these professionals are "not adequately trained to provide proper assessment, treatment, and management of suicidal clients; or to know how to refer them properly for specialized assessment and treatment." In fact, studies indicate that 90% of those who die by suicide had a diagnosable Axis I disorder (Conwell et al., 1996) and that many clients had contact with a mental health professional during the final year of their lives (Luoma, Martin, & Pearson, 2002). In their meta-analysis, Luoma and colleagues found that approximately one-fifth of those who died by suicide (19%) had contact with a mental health professional within 1 month of their suicide and approximately one-third (32%) had such contact within 1 year of their suicide.

There is no question that adequate training for mental health professionals is one key suicide prevention strategy. With funding from the DHHS, the "Core Competencies" initiative was spearheaded by the Suicide Prevention Resource Center in collaboration with the American Association of Suicidology. A team of professionals reviewed the evidence base and reached a consensus on core competencies for training purposes. This team included Lanny Berman, Thomas Ellis, Nadine Kaslow, David Rudd, Shawn Shea, Marsha Linehan, Rheeda Walker, David Litts, Xan Young, and one of the authors of this book, Cheryl A. King. Twenty-four core competencies were established; eight of these were designated as the core competencies for the 1-day workshop, "Assessing and Managing Suicide Risk" (Suicide Prevention Resource Center, 2008), and all 24 were designated as the training competencies for the 2-day workshop, "Recognizing and Responding to Suicide Risk," sponsored by the American Association of Suicidology. The eight core competencies, essential to practice with a suicidal individual, include:

- Managing one's reactions to suicide.
- Reconciling the difference (and potential conflict) between the clinician's goal to prevent suicide and the client's goal to eliminate psychological pain.
- Maintaining a collaborative, nonadversarial stance.
- Eliciting suicide ideation, behavior, plans, and intent.
- Making a clinical judgment of the risk that a client will attempt or complete suicide in the short and long term.
- Collaboratively developing a crisis response plan.
- Developing a written treatment and services plan that addresses the client's immediate, acute, and continuing suicide ideation and risk for suicide behaviors.
- Developing policies and procedures for following clients closely, including taking reasonable steps to be proactive.

This practitioner guide builds on this core competencies approach and carefully considers and incorporates many of the recommendations from published guidelines.

CONCLUSION

In this practitioner guide, we present the core knowledge, competencies, and skills that are essential to effective, evidence-based practice with suicidal teens. Specifically, we focus on evidence-based screening, risk assessment and formulation, and care management. This book brings together in one accessible guide the essential information, real-world examples, and useful clinical tools.

CHAPTER TWO

A Look at Overall Risk and Protective Factors

▶ Define risk and protective factors.

▶ Review risk factors for suicide attempts and suicide, including:

  ▪ Demographics;

  ▪ Clinical characteristics;

  ▪ Contextual/interpersonal factors.

▶ Discuss connectedness as a possible protective factor for suicide attempts and suicide.

In this chapter, we examine factors that may either contribute to or protect adolescents from suicide risk. We begin by defining risk and protective factors. We then provide you with a current evidence-based review of these factors as they relate to adolescent suicidal behavior and suicide. As a result, this is the most "research-heavy" chapter within this book. We believe this foundation of knowledge will enable you to be more confident in your screening, risk assessment, and ultimately your decision making about how best to prevent suicidal behavior in at-risk adolescents.

In subsequent chapters, we refer back to the information provided here and describe how these factors may guide our decisions about the acuity of risk, need to hospitalize, and crisis response planning.

WHAT ARE RISK AND PROTECTIVE FACTORS?

Suicide risk factors are characteristics that *precede the suicidal behavior or suicide* and that *increase the likelihood of suicidal behavior or suicide*. They are well-defined constructs, based on empirical evidence (Rudd et al., 2006). It is important to keep in mind that risk factors are population dependent; in other words, studies may identify one constellation of risk factors for young people and a somewhat different pattern of risk factors for elderly adults. Furthermore, a risk factor may have a different impact depending on many important considerations, including duration of exposure to the risk factor, when the exposure occurred (e.g., at what age), and the intensity of the risk factor (Costello, Angold, Cicchetti, & Cohen, 2006). In other words, knowing the research evidence is necessary, but not sufficient. We must always view each teen as an individual and consider the unique aspects of his or her situation.

Protective factors are variables that *decrease the probability of suicidal behavior and suicide*. For example, research studies indicate that strong problem-solving skills and social connectedness may function as protective factors. It is important to note that, although there is a large body of converging evidence about risk factors for adolescent suicide, we have less information about protective factors. This is partially because much of the research on teen suicidal behavior and suicide has focused on identifying factors that increase risk, whereas relatively little has focused on what protects against suicide or how to most effectively intervene. In addition, many protective factors may be far upstream from suicidal behavior and suicide. These might be factors such as a secure and safe childhood that protects against physical and sexual abuse, the development of strong coping and problem-solving skills, and residence in a home and community that minimizes the likelihood of alcohol and drug abuse. These protective factors may occur early in life and continue throughout development. Rather than specifically protecting against suicide, they protect against many adverse outcomes.

HOW DO WE CONCEPTUALIZE RISK FACTORS?

Risk factors can be characterized as either *acute* or *chronic*. As one example, a teen with a psychiatric disorder such as major depressive disorder or bipolar disorder may be at acute risk when there is a crisis or negative life change (e.g., a relationship breakup or disciplinary action) that increases the chance of suicidal behavior. Acute risk is thought to be time limited; however, it can last from minutes to hours to days (Bryan & Rudd, 2006) and frequently occurs in someone with one or more chronic risk factors. Chronic risk factors place teens at elevated risk for a lengthy period of time. A teen with a long history of impulsivity and substance abuse may be at chronic risk for suicide. It is important to note that teens at chronic risk for suicide may experience a crisis and be at particularly high risk due to the combination of chronic and acute risk factors. Some experts would define this as "chronic high risk with acute exacerbation" (Bryan & Rudd, 2006). Acute risk factors are often described as "warning signs" for exacerbated suicide risk.

Some risk factors are static, or *nonmodifiable*, meaning that they cannot be changed. An example would be a childhood history of sexual abuse. Nonmodifiable risk factors are important because they help us understand why some teens may have chronic or lifelong elevated suicide risk. Other risk factors are *modifiable*. These conditions can be changed and may be the targets of intervention. An example would be depressed mood, which we would hope to modify or improve with treatment. Risk factors can also be thought of as *proximal or distal*. Proximal risk factors are closely linked in time to the suicide event or may even act as a trigger (Moscicki,

1995). Two of the most common proximal risk factors—precipitants of adolescent suicidal behavior—are relationship breakups or conflicts and disciplinary actions (Brent, Perper, Moritz, & Baugher, 1993a). Distal risk factors have usually occurred in the past, but nevertheless continue to exert an influence on suicide risk. For example, a distal risk factor may be sexual abuse that occurred 3 years ago, with the proximal risk factor being a recent breakup with a boyfriend.

RISK FACTORS FOR TEEN SUICIDE AND SUICIDAL BEHAVIOR

In this chapter, we categorize the risk factors pertinent to comprehensive risk assessments into three groups: demographic features, clinical features, and family and interpersonal factors. A one-page information sheet for use as a reference in your practice is included in **Appendix A**, **Risk Factor Checklist for Teen Suicidal Behavior and Suicide**. In Chapter 4, we describe how to use the information on risk factors to conduct an evidence-based risk assessment with a teen.

Demographic Features

Gender

Among teens, males are more likely to die by suicide than females (CDC, 2012a). As is evident in Table 2.1, the ratio of male to female suicide increases across the teenage years. By age 19, the prevalence rate of suicide for males is more than five times greater than the rate for females.

This gender difference in suicide prevalence rates may be partially due to the method of attempt. Among boys ages 15–19 years, the most common method is a firearm. Among girls ages 10–19 years and boys ages 10–14 years, the most common method is hanging and suffocation. Historically and at this time, teenage boys have been much more likely to use a highly lethal method such

TABLE 2.1. Suicide Deaths per 100,000 Teens in the United States, 2002–2009

	\multicolumn{7}{c}{Age in years}						
	13	14	15	16	17	18	19
Males	2.2	3.5	5.8	8.5	11.2	15.0	18.3
Females	1.0	1.7	2.5	2.9	2.9	2.8	3.4

Note. Adapted from CDC (2012a).

as firearms when attempting suicide. However, it is important to note that in recent years, the prevalence of suicide by hanging and suffocation has increased among teenage girls. This is a disturbing trend due to the associated lethality. Among girls ages 10–14 years, hanging and suffocation accounted for 0.15 deaths per 100,000 in 1990 and 0.72 deaths per 100,000 in 2009. Among girls ages 15–19 years, the rates increased from 0.55 to 1.86 deaths per 100,000 over the same span. When an adolescent has made a previous suicide attempt, information about the method is an important consideration in the risk assessment and formulation.

As indicated in Table 2.2, the prevalence rate for suicide *attempts* follows a different gender pattern than the rate for suicide. Girls are more likely to attempt suicide than boys. Rates of suicide

TABLE 2.2. Summary of U.S. National Prevalence Data for Demographic Risk Factors

Age	Older teens and young adults are more likely to die by suicide than younger teens.
	In contrast, suicide attempts are less likely during the late teen and young adult years than during the middle teen years.
Gender	Boys are more likely to die by suicide than girls.
	Girls are more likely to attempt suicide than boys.
Race	American Indian and Alaskan Native adolescents are at highest risk for suicide and suicide attempts.
	African American teens have lower rates of suicide than do Caucasian and Hispanic teens.

Note. Adapted from CDC (2012a).

attempt are actually one and a half to two times higher for female teenagers (9.8%) compared to their male peers (5.8%) (CDC, 2012b).

Age

Suicide rates increase across childhood and adolescence. In fact, suicide is actually quite rare before the age of 9 years, accounting for far fewer than 1 death per 100,000 children in a given year (CDC, 2012a). The rate increases only slightly from ages 10 to 14 years (1.17 deaths per 100,000), making it the third leading cause of death following accidents and cancer.

The most dramatic increase in suicide occurs during the teenage years. Only death by accidents and homicide outnumber those by suicide in the 15-to-19-year-old age group within the United States, with suicide accounting for 7.47 deaths per 100,000 in 2009. Beginning at age 14, suicide becomes the second leading cause of death. It remains the second leading cause until the age of 17, when the prevalence of homicide surpasses the prevalence of suicide (CDC, 2012a).

Suicide attempt rates do not show the same clear pattern of increase across the adolescent years. The Youth Risk Behavior Surveillance examined the self-reported suicide attempts of high school students in 2011. The percentage of teenagers attempting suicide was higher among 9th-grade (9.3%), 10th-grade (8.2%), and 11th-grade (6.6%) students than among 12th-grade (6.3%) students (CDC, 2012b). There is a tapering of suicide attempt behavior across late adolescence and early adulthood, a period when the prevalence of death by suicide is increasing. This pattern of differing prevalence rates across adolescents and young adulthood is summarized in Table 2.2. It suggests the importance of identifying and intervening as early as possible with the suicidal or potentially suicidal teenager.

Race/Ethnicity

Suicide rates in teenagers (15–19 years old) vary by race and ethnicity. One of the most striking findings is the suicide rate for

American Indian and Alaskan Natives. Among these teens, rates are more than 2.3 times that of non-Hispanic Caucasians (20.7 vs. 8.9 per 100,000, respectively). The rates of suicide among other racial/ethnic groups are as follows: Caucasians (8.4 per 100,000), Asian/Pacific Islanders (5.9), Hispanic Caucasians (6.3) and Blacks (4.4) (CDC, 2012a).

Suicide *attempts* follow a slightly different racial and ethnic pattern. In concordance with the suicide rate, American Indian adolescents have the highest suicide *attempt* rate (see Table 2.2). However, Hispanics have the next highest rate followed by Blacks, Caucasian, and Asian American adolescents (CDC, 2012b).

Demographic risk factors are especially important when designing large-scale public health approaches to adolescent suicide prevention because they guide decisions about where to allocate the most resources. *When working with individual teens, one must be cautious about overinterpreting findings that are based on large groups of individuals.* Indeed, despite the relatively low prevalence rate for suicide among the U.S. population of teenage girls, especially Black teenage girls, an individual Black teenage girl may be highly suicidal and must be taken seriously and evaluated carefully. Clinicians should view demographic risk factors as just one piece of information in a comprehensive risk assessment (described in Chapter 4).

CLINICAL NOTE

1. Suicide attempts and suicides occur among male and female teens of all ages and all racial/ethnic groups.

2. In a clinical setting, individual clinical and family/interpersonal risk factors take precedence over demographic risk factors when evaluating risk.

3. When engaged in larger-scale public health preventive strategies, demographic risk factors point us to high-risk subgroups.

Clinical Features

Risk factors categorized as individual clinical features include characteristics of the teen (e.g., suicide attempt history, psychiatric condition, mental status) and recent discharge from a psychiatric hospital. These are outlined in Table 2.3. Moreover, in Chapter 4 and in **Appendix E, Teen Suicide Risk Assessment Worksheet**, we provide a structured form for interviewers to use as a tool in gathering this information.

Previous Suicide Attempt

One of the strongest predictors of suicide in teens is a past suicide attempt. Approximately 40% of young people who die by suicide have made a prior suicide attempt (Brent, Kolko, Wartella, &

TABLE 2.3. Individual Clinical Risk Factors

History of suicide attempt
  Multiple past attempts associated with highest risk

Suicidal ideation and intent

Psychiatric disorders
  Depressive or bipolar disorder
  Alcohol/drug abuse
  Conduct disorder/disruptive behavior disorders
  Posttraumatic stress disorder
  Other (anxiety disorder, eating disorder, schizophrenia)

Other behaviors and characteristics
  Nonsuicidal self-injury
  Emerging personality disorder traits
    Cluster B (dramatic, emotional)
    Cluster C (anxious, fearful)
  Hopelessness
  Impulsivity
  Aggressiveness/history of violent behavior
  Sleep disturbance
  Learning disorders and difficulties

Discharge from psychiatric hospital

Boylan, 1993; Brent, Perper, Moritz, Allman, et al., 1993; Shaffer, Gould, Fisher, & Trautman, 1996). Even when we take into account depressive symptoms, a history of suicide attempts remains significant as a predictor (Lewinsohn, Rohde, & Seeley, 1994). Risk increases further with the number of previous attempts. Teenagers with multiple past attempts are twice as likely to make another attempt compared to those teens with no attempts or only one previous attempt (Goldston et al., 1999).

Suicidal Ideation and Intent

Suicidal thoughts are common among adolescents. As noted in Chapter 1, nationally representative studies indicate that 15.8% of high school students have seriously considered making a suicide attempt within the past 12 months and 12.8% of high school students report that they have made a plan about how they would attempt suicide (CDC, 2012b). The presence, frequency, and severity of suicidal ideation are all predictive of a later suicide attempt. For example, in one large community-based study, 88% of teenage suicide attempters reported having had suicidal thoughts prior to their suicide attempt (Lewinsohn, Rohde, & Seeley, 1996). Mild and infrequent suicidal thoughts were associated with a 2.8% likelihood of a suicide attempt in the following year, whereas more severe and frequent suicidal thoughts were associated with a 16.7% likelihood of a suicide attempt in the next year (Lewinsohn et al., 1996). The "take-home message" from these statistics is that even mild and infrequent thoughts of suicide should be taken seriously, as they convey increased risk for a suicide attempt.

Nonsuicidal Self-Injury

Nonsuicidal self-injury (NSSI) refers to the "intentional destruction of body tissue without suicidal intent and for purposes not socially sanctioned" (Klonsky, 2007). Common forms of NSSI are skin cutting, scratching, burning, and banging or hitting. Such behaviors are deliberate, usually begin in early adolescence, and are reported by 15% to 25% of high school students (Muehlenkamp & Gutierrez,

2004, 2007). Not surprisingly, NSSI is reported by an even higher percentage of adolescents in clinical settings. These adolescents have been found to meet diagnostic criteria for a wide range of disorders, including internalizing disorders, externalizing disorders, personality disorders, and alcohol/substance use disorders (Nock, Joiner, Gordon, Lloyd-Richardson, & Prinstein, 2006).

The function of NSSI can be differentiated from the function of suicide attempts. Whereas the function of NSSI is often to manage or regulate emotions—particularly strong negative emotions—the function of a suicide attempt is clearly not to feel better and improve one's life. As discussed by Klonsky (2007), converging evidence from multiple studies indicates that NSSI is associated with decreases in negative affect and arousal and with the experience of relief. Other functions of NSSI that have received some empirical support include, among others, self-punishment, an effort to influence others, and sensation seeking.

NSSI suggests elevated risk of suicidal behavior and, in fact, NSSI and suicide attempt behavior often co-occur. In a community sample, approximately 50% of adolescents who engaged in NSSI also reported at least one suicide attempt (Muehlenkamp & Gutierrez, 2007). In a sample of adolescents on a psychiatric inpatient unit who had engaged in NSSI, 70% reported a history of at least one suicide attempt and 55% reported a history of multiple suicide attempts (Nock et al., 2006). Moreover, among depressed adolescents, NSSI has been associated with increased risk of a suicide attempt and has functioned as a stronger predictor of a new suicide attempt than has a prior suicide attempt (Asarnow et al., 2011; Wilkinson, Kelvin, Roberts, Dubicka, & Goodyer, 2011).

Among adolescents who engage in NSSI, indicators of increased risk of suicide attempt may include a negative attitude toward life (Muehlenkamp & Gutierrez, 2004), lower self-esteem, less parental support, and greater suicidal ideation (Brausch & Gutierrez, 2010). Other risk factors are a more chronic history of NSSI and using a variety of methods to engage in NSSI (Nock et al., 2006). These findings underscore the importance of further assessing all self-harmful behaviors and conducting comprehensive risk assessments, whether suicidal intent is present.

21

Psychiatric Disorders/Psychopathology

A psychiatric disorder is one of the most common risk factors for suicide in teenagers. We have learned from psychological autopsy studies that approximately 90% of teenagers who died by suicide had at least one psychiatric disorder (Brent, Perper, Moritz, Allman, et al., 1993; Marttunen, Aro, Henriksson, & Lonnqvist, 1991; Shaffer, Gould, Fisher, & Trautman, 1996; Shafii, Steltz-Lenarsky, Derrick, & Beckner, 1988) at the time of their death and many had more than one psychiatric condition (Shaffer et al., 1996; Shafii et al., 1988).

Older teenagers with multiple psychiatric disorders and teenagers with an early onset of psychiatric disorders are at especially high risk. For instance, the combination of psychiatric disorder and substance abuse is both more common and associated with a higher risk for suicide in older versus younger adolescents (Brent, Baugher, Bridge, Chen, & Chiappetta, 1999).

Depressive Disorders. Depressive disorders are well established as a risk factor for suicidal behavior (Beautrais, Joyce, Mulder, & Fergusson, 1996), repeat attempts (Goldston et al., 1998), and suicide (Brent, Perper, Moritz, Allman, et al., 1993; Goldston et al., 1999; Shaffer et al., 1996). Approximately 50 to 60% of adolescents who die by suicide have a mood disorder (Marttunen et al., 1991; Shaffer et al., 1996). Furthermore, suicidal ideation is a frequently occurring symptom in adolescents with major depressive disorder (MDD). In a longitudinal study, Myers, McCauley, Calderon, and Treder (1991) found that 72% of those with MDD reported suicidal thoughts or behaviors across a 3-year period.

Bipolar Disorder. Bipolar disorder (BP) is associated with elevated risk of suicidal behavior and suicide. Converging evidence from several research studies supports this finding. In a naturalistic, prospective follow-up of 54 adolescents with bipolar disorder who were psychiatrically hospitalized, Strober and colleagues (Strober, Schmidt-Lackner, Freeman, & Bower, 1995) reported that 20% of these adolescents had made severe, medically significant suicide attempts. In a longer, 10-year follow-up, Welner and colleagues (Welner, Welner, & Fishman, 1979) reported that 25% of adolescents with BP who had been psychiatrically hospitalized eventually died by suicide. In a clinical study of 405 children and adolescents who met DSM-IV criteria for BP (BPI, BPII, or BP NOS), Goldstein and colleagues (2005) reported that 32% of these patients endorsed at least one suicide attempt. In this study, there were multiple key predictors of history of suicide attempt: mixed episodes, psychiatric hospitalization, history of self-injurious behavior, substance use disorder, and panic disorder. Finally, case–control studies of adolescents who have died by suicide indicate that BP is associated with an elevated risk for suicide (Brent et al., 1988; Brent, Perper, Moritz, Allman, et al., 1993).

Alcohol and Drug Abuse. Alcohol and drug abuse significantly increases the risk for suicide (Brent, Perper, Moritz, Allman, et al., 1993; Marttunen et al., 1991; Shafii et al., 1988), perhaps because of the associated decrease in inhibition and problems in adaptive functioning. Marttunen and colleagues (1991) reported that 51% of teens who died by suicide had consumed alcohol before their death and many were intoxicated at the time of death, making alcohol use a proximal risk factor for suicidal behavior.

The risk of suicidal behavior increases as substance use transitions into substance abuse; studies have focused on alcohol, cannabis, and other substances (Beautrais, Joyce, & Mulder, 1996; Groves, Stanley, & Sher, 2007). Studies estimate that male adolescents with alcohol dependence are 15 times more likely to attempt suicide and female adolescents are three times more likely to attempt suicide (Esposito-Smythers & Spirito, 2004). This risk is even higher when a substance use disorder is comorbid with an affective disorder (Brent, Perper, Moritz, Allman, et al., 1993; Wagner, Cole, & Schwartzman, 1996).

High-risk behaviors among teens, such as alcohol and drug use, multiple sexual partners, sex for drugs or money, and IV drug use, have been closely examined in relation to depression, suicidal ideation, and previous suicide attempts, using data from the National Longitudinal Study of Adolescent Health (Add Health; Hallfors et al., 2004). In this nationally representative sample, membership in multiple high-risk behavior clusters was associated with suicidal ideation and a history of suicide attempt. However, membership in the "increasingly deviant risk clusters," including the use of marijuana and other illegal drugs, was associated with a particularly high likelihood of a suicide attempt. More recently, Pena, Matthieu, Zayas, Maysn, and Caine (2012) examined data from five national administrations of the Youth Risk Behavior Surveillance System (1999 to 2007), identifying 1,395 adolescents who reported a suicide attempt during the past year for which they received medical attention. These investigators found that the probability of multiple suicide attempts increased as the severity of substance abuse and violent behaviors increased. Substance abuse and other high risk-behaviors are clearly associated with increased risk of suicide attempt.

Conduct Disorder, Disruptive Behavior Disorders, and Impulse Control Problems. Disruptive behavior disorders, including conduct disorder, are also a risk factor for adolescent suicide. Approximately 20 to 50% of adolescents who die by suicide have some type of conduct or disruptive disorder, which is commonly comorbid with mood, anxiety, or substance abuse disorders (Brent, Perper, Moritz, Allman, et al., 1993; Marttunen et al., 1991; Shaffer et al., 1996). Conduct disorder remains an important risk factor even in the absence of a mood disorder (Brent, Perper, Moritz, Allman, et al., 1993). The risk for suicide *attempt* is also increased in the presence of conduct and antisocial disorders (Beautrais, Joyce, et al., 1996).

Impulse control problems are often a hallmark of disruptive behavior disorders, and it may be the symptom of impulsivity that increases suicide risk. Impulsivity has been associated with suicidal behavior in numerous clinical studies (Horesh, Gothelf, Ofek, Weizman, & Apter, 1999; Kashden, Fremouw, Callahan, & Franzen, 1993).

Posttraumatic Stress Disorder and Other Anxiety Disorders. Posttraumatic stress disorder (PTSD) is strongly associated with adolescent suicide attempts (Giaconia, Reinherz, Silverman, & Pakiz, 1995). In one study of 3,021 adolescents and young adults ages 14–24 years, those suffering from PTSD were found to have the greatest increased risk for suicide attempt, relative to those with other anxiety, depressive, substance use, and eating disorders (Wunderlich, Bronisch, & Wittchen, 1998). Young adults who were exposed to trauma and developed PTSD were significantly more likely to attempt suicide compared to those exposed to a trauma who did not develop PTSD (Wilcox, Storr, & Breslau, 2009). This association was consistent regardless of the type of trauma (e.g., combat trauma, sexual abuse, natural disaster; Panagioti, Gooding, & Tarrier, 2009).

Evidence is mixed regarding the relationship between other types of anxiety and risk for suicide. Some studies suggest that anxiety, broadly defined, is associated with elevated risk for adolescent suicide attempts (Gould et al., 1998; Wunderlich et al., 1998), whereas others suggest that after comorbid depressive disorders are taken into account, suicidal adolescents are not more likely to have an anxiety disorder diagnosis. When anxiety disorders have been identified in the histories of adolescents who have died by suicide, these disorders have generally been comorbid with affective disorders (Brent, Perper, Moritz, Allman, et al., 1993). Although findings are mixed (Andrews & Lewinsohn, 1992; Gould et al., 1998; Pilowsky, Wu, & Anthony, 1999), at least one study (Pilowsky et al., 1999), reported that adolescents experiencing panic attacks were two times more likely than their peers to attempt suicide.

Eating Disorders and Body Image Disorders. Adolescents who engage in extreme weight control behaviors are at higher risk for suicide attempts than other adolescents (Neumark-Sztainer, Story, Dixon, & Murray, 1998). Similarly, body image is related to suicide attempts. A community sample of middle school students in eastern North Carolina showed that girls were more likely to attempt suicide if they perceived themselves as being overweight. In this same sample, boys were more likely to attempt suicide if they perceived themselves as being either over- or underweight (Whetstone, Morrissey, & Cummings, 2007).

Schizophrenia. Schizophrenia is relatively rare among adolescents and does not account for a significant percentage of suicides in this age group. Nevertheless, the early course of illness in schizophrenia has been conceptualized as a deterioration phase, and several studies have reported a particularly high risk for suicide among young adults with schizophrenia (early in the course of illness; Palmer, Pankratz, & Bostwick, 2005). Reporting on a nationwide psychological autopsy study of 92 suicide victims with schizophrenia in Finland, Heila and colleagues (1997) noted that 7% of the overall group of individuals who died by suicide had suffered with schizophrenia. Although the mean age of these individuals was 40 years, the authors reported that the age range for the suicides was 16 to 77 years.

Emerging Personality Disorder Traits

Personality disorders are not generally diagnosed in children and adolescents under 18 years (American Psychiatric Association, 2000); however, it is not uncommon in clinical practice to observe personality disorder traits among adolescents. In fact, several studies support a relationship between emerging personality disorder and adolescent suicide (Brent, Johnson, et al., 1993; Brent, Johnson, et al., 1994; Pfeffer, Newcorn, Kaplan, & Mizruchi, 1988). Rates for personality disorder in adolescents who die by suicide have been reported to be approximately 30% (Marttunen et al., 1991; Shafii et al., 1988); Cluster B (dramatic, emotional, or erratic disorders), followed by Cluster C (anxious or fearful disorders) personality traits are the most common of the Axis II disorders reported in suicidal adolescents (Brent, Johnson, et al., 1993).

Hopelessness

Conceptualized as negative expectations about the future, hopelessness is often considered in conjunction with depressive symptoms and disorders. Nevertheless, hopelessness may also contribute independently to suicide risk. It has been related to suicidal ideation, suicidal intent, and suicide attempts in both community-based samples (e.g, Mazza & Reynolds, 1998) and clinical samples (e.g., Reinecke, DuBois, & Schultz, 2001). Hopelessness has also been related to future suicide attempts (Goldston et al., 2001). As such, an assessment of hopelessness is an important component to a careful suicide risk formulation. Hopelessness is also particularly important to assess because it may be a modifiable risk factor. Many cognitive therapy approaches are designed to reframe adolescents' negative or maladaptive thought patterns. Addressing hopelessness, especially about the possible benefit of treatment, is a critical first step to securing adolescent buy-in for treatment.

Learning Disorders and Difficulties

Recent research has documented a link between increased risk for suicide attempts and suicide with learning disorders and untreated learning difficulties (Bender, Rosenkrans, & Crane, 1999; Daniel et al., 2006). In particular, students who are failing, or even perceive themselves to be experiencing academic failure, are at increased risk for suicide. Often these students may have untreated attention or learning problems that have reduced their academic self-esteem and may be contributing to their mood difficulties. When the teen is stable, having him or her undergo a thorough psychoeducational or neuropsychological evaluation can be helpful and may suggest other more appropriate educational interventions for the future.

Sleep Disturbance

It is well known that irregular sleep patterns, often characterized by staying up late and sleeping in, are relatively common among adolescents, and that significant numbers of teens struggle with sleep deprivation and daytime sleepiness (e.g., McKnight-Eily et al., 2011). There is also evidence to suggest that adolescents are particularly vulnerable to sleep disturbances such as insomnia (Roane & Taylor, 2008). Converging evidence has established a relation between sleep disturbance and both suicidal ideation and suicide attempts in adolescents (e.g., Liu, 2004; Roane & Taylor, 2008). As examples, using data from the National Longitudinal Study of Adolescent Health

(Add Health) in the United States, Roane and Taylor reported that 9.4% of adolescents experienced symptoms of insomnia. These symptoms were associated with alcohol and substance abuse, depression, suicidal ideation, and suicide attempts. Similarly, McKnight-Eily et al. (2011) examined associations between inadequate sleep (less than 8 hours on school nights) and health risk behaviors such as cigarette smoking, substance abuse, physical fighting, low levels of physical activity, and seriously considering making a suicide attempt. These investigators reported that inadequate sleep was associated with multiple health risk behaviors, including seriously considering making a suicide attempt. Finally, Goldstein, Bridge, and Brent (2008) used the psychological autopsy method to examine sleep disturbances in 140 adolescents who died by suicide and in a control group of adolescents. The adolescents who died by suicide were five times more likely to have struggled with insomnia in the week prior to their death, even after controlling for depression severity.

Discharge from a Psychiatric Hospital

A heightened time of concern for suicide attempts among adolescents is the period after discharge from an inpatient psychiatric hospitalization. Studies indicate that 10–18% of adolescents attempt suicide during the 6 months following psychiatric hospitalization (Brent, Kolko, et al., 1993; King, Segal, Kaminski, & Naylor, 1995). Furthermore, in a 5-year follow-up study, the period of highest risk was during the first year after discharge, with 12% of the total sample making an attempt, including 7.8% of adolescents with no previous attempt (Goldston et al., 1999).

Family and Interpersonal Factors

Family and interpersonal risk factors include family characteristics and the nature of the adolescent's social relationships and interactions with others. These factors may consist of a parent who has died by suicide, low levels of perceived peer support, a history of abuse or bullying, or struggles with sexual identity.

Family Psychiatric History

Adolescents are at higher risk for suicidal behavior and suicide if they have a family member who has struggled with suicidal behavior. More specifically, adolescent suicide is five times more likely in the offspring of mothers and twice as likely in the offspring of fathers who died by suicide even after adjusting for the parents' psychiatric diagnoses (Agerbo, Nordentoft, & Mortensen, 2002). Twin studies suggest that the suicide risk has some element of heritability that is independent of the family environment (Heath et al., 2002; McGuffin, Marusic, & Farmer, 2001).

Family psychiatric disorders are also likely to affect suicidal behavior in young people. First-degree relatives with antisocial personality disorder (Brent et al., 1988; Pfeffer, Normandin, & Kakuma, 1994), substance abuse disorders (Pfeffer et al., 1994), and affective disorders (Brent et al., 1988; Brent, Perper, Moritz, & Liotus, 1994) increase the risk for adolescent suicidal behavior. Parental psychopathology may affect adolescents in a number of ways, for example, via increased biological/genetic risk for the same illness, via parenting impairments that are secondary to the parents' illness, or via increased environmental stressors that are secondary to parent mental health problems, to name a few possible pathways.

Sexual Abuse

Multiple studies have documented an association between sexual abuse and increased suicide risk for both teenage boys and girls. Studies of nationally representative samples (e.g., Martin, Bergen, Richardson, Roeger, & Allison, 2004) show that teenagers reporting a history of sexual abuse are more likely (24%) than their non-abused peers (5%) to attempt suicide. Of even more concern is that many of these abused adolescents make several suicide attempts (Belik, Cox, Stein, Asmundson, & Sareen, 2007; Martin et al., 2004; Sigfusdottir, Asgeirsdottir, Gudjonsson, & Sigurdsson, 2008).

Physical Abuse and Neglect

Physical abuse and neglect are associated with both suicide (Brent, Perper, Moritz, & Baugher, 1993b; Shafii, Carrigan, Whittinghill, & Derrick, 1985) and suicidal behavior (Borowsky, Resnick, Ireland, & Blum, 1999; Grossman, Milligan, & Deyo, 1991; Salzinger, Ng-Mak, Rosario, & Feldman, 2007). This association is robust and thought to cross racial and ethnic lines (King & Merchant, 2008). Few studies look at neglect separately from physical abuse; however, Arata and colleagues (Arata, Langhinrichsen-Rohling, Bowers, & O'Brien, 2007) showed that neglect alone predicted higher levels of suicide risk (risk taking and suicide-related behaviors) than did physical abuse or sexual abuse in a large community sample of adolescents.

Bullying/Peer Victimization

Bullying, also referred to as peer victimization, has been linked to an increased likelihood of suicidal ideation and suicide attempts in multiple studies (Baldry & Winkel, 2003; Delfabbro et al., 2006; Liang, Flisher, & Lombard, 2007; Park, Schepp, Jang, & Koo, 2006; Toros, Bilgin, Sasmaz, Bugdayci, & Camdeviren, 2004). Russell and Joyner (2001) examined data from a large nationally representative study in the United States, the National Longitudinal Study of Adolescent Health (Add Health). After taking into account the effects of sexual orientation, hopelessness, depression, alcohol abuse, and family/friend history of suicidal ideation and behavior, adolescents who reported histories of victimization were more likely to report suicidal thoughts and attempts. Similarly, in a clinical sample of youth admitted to the hospital after a suicide attempt, Davies and Cunningham (1999) found that being bullied contributed to the suicide attempts of 22% of these youth. In summary, the findings of research studies converge to indicate that peer victimization is a significant predictor of suicidal ideation and suicide attempts.

Studies conducted in multiple nations have reported similar findings. In their study of 998 youth from schools in Rome, Baldry and Winkel (2003) found that direct (physical, psychological, or verbal bullying) and relational (social exclusion, malicious rumor spreading) victimization were correlated with suicidal ideation. These investigators found that, after taking into account the effects of physical harm from parents, domestic violence between parents, and demographic variables, only relational victimization predicted suicidal ideation. These findings underscore the importance of social exclusion or "thwarted belongingness" as a risk factor.

Interestingly, it is not only the targets of peer victimization who are at increased risk for suicide and suicidal behaviors (Klomek, Marrocco, Kleinman, Schonfeld, & Gould, 2007; Roland, 2002). Bullies have also been shown to be at increased risk for suicide-related outcomes. In a Finnish sample of adolescents ages 14–16 years, both bullies and those who were bullied had an increased risk of depression and suicidal ideation. Furthermore, bullies were as depressed as those who were bullied, and, after accounting for depression, suicidal ideation was more common among bullies (Kaltiala-Heino, Rimpelä, Marttunen, Rimpelä, & Rantanen, 1999).

Peer Relationships

In addition to peer victimization and the perpetration of bullying, the quality of a teen's relationships with peers is important to consider when determining suicide risk status (King & Merchant, 2008). As an example, Johnson and colleagues (2002) conducted a longitudinal study of 659 families from northern New York. After taking into account age, gender, psychiatric symptoms, and parental psychiatric symptoms, they found a wide range of interpersonal difficulties that were associated with risk for suicide attempts. These included difficulty making friends, frequent cruelty toward peers, frequent refusal to share, frequent arguments or anger with peers, social isolation, lack of close friends, and poor relationships with friends and peers. Perceived peer rejection and low levels of friendship support also have been directly associated with higher levels of suicidal ideation among adolescents (Prinstein, Boergers, Spirito, Little, & Grapentine, 2000).

Family Characteristics

In addition to family psychiatric history, risk for suicidal behavior among adolescents may be related to family characteristics such as family attachment, perceived family support, parent–adolescent communication, and parent–child conflict (King & Merchant, 2008).

Community studies document associations between low family support and both suicidal ideation and suicide attempts among adolescents (Dubow, Kausch, Blum, Reed, & Bush, 1989; Perkins & Hartless, 2002). Furthermore, in a prospective community-based study of depressed adolescents, low social support from family predicted suicide attempts in adulthood for females (Lewinsohn, Rohde, Seeley, & Baldwin, 2001). Similarly, poor attachment with the parent is associated with suicide attempts (Fergusson, Woodward, & Horwood, 2000), and teenagers from families with more conflict or discord (Asarnow, Carlson, & Guthrie, 1987; Pfeffer, Klerman, Hurt, & Kakuma, 1993) and lower levels of perceived family support (Lewinsohn et al., 1994; O'Donnell, Stueve, Wardlaw, & O'Donnell, 2003) are more likely to attempt suicide. Furthermore, teens who die by suicide are more likely to have had less frequent and less satisfying communication with their parents (Gould, Fisher, Parides, Flory, & Shaffer, 1996).

In a clinical study, suicidal adolescent inpatients with mood disorders have reported lower levels of support from their families than nonsuicidal adolescent inpatients with mood disorders (King, Segal, Naylor, & Evans, 1993). Moreover, research indicates that suicidal adolescents reporting less family support are also more likely to attempt suicide during the 6 months following their psychiatric hospitalization (King et al., 1995). Adolescents' perceptions of support or connectedness may be a more powerful predictor of mood and functioning than objective measures of support. For example, Cumsille and Epstein (1994) found that satisfaction with family functioning was the strongest predictor of depression in adolescents. This suggests the importance of measuring subjective perceptions of social connections.

Adolescents who live in families that move a lot may also be at increased risk for suicide. Brent, Perper, et al. (1994) examined this issue and found that adolescents who died by suicide were more likely to have had residential instability compared to demographically matched controls. Another interesting finding is that moving one's family residence had a greater impact on girls, who were approximately 60% more likely to report a suicide attempt during the following year. In this same study, there was no association between moving and suicide attempts for boys (Haynie, South, & Bose, 2006). It is important to note that a third variable, such as problem behaviors or a lack of friendships, may have accounted for moves and served to increase the risk for suicidal behavior, rather than the residential instability.

Sexual Orientation and Identity

The rates of suicidal ideation and attempt are reported to be higher in adolescents who identify themselves as lesbian, gay, bisexual, or transgender (LGBT). Approximately 30% of LGBT youth attempt suicide at least once (D'Augelli, Hershberger, & Pilkington, 2001; Garofalo, Wolf, Wissow, Woods, & Goodman, 1999; Remafedi, French, Story, Resnick, & Blum, 1998). Among these, approximately half have reported that the suicide attempt was related to their sexual orientation (D'Augelli et al., 2001). Rates for suicide attempt in this population are commonly higher for male teenagers compared to their female peers. Factors associated with LGBT-related suicide attempts include early openness about sexual orientation, being considered gender atypical in childhood by parents, and parental efforts to discourage gender atypical behaviors (D'Augelli et al., 2005). In a recent longitudinal study of specific risk factors in LGBT youth, ages 16-20 years, a history of suicide attempt, impulsive behavior, LGBT victimization, and low social support were associated with greater suicidal ideation (Liu & Mustanski, 2012).

Contextual Factors

Exposure to Suicide

Suicide occurring in clusters is also known as a contagion. It is well documented across cultures that adolescents are at increased risk for suicide after being exposed to a suicide (Brent, Kerr, Goldstein, & Bozigar, 1989; Gould, Wallenstein, & Kleinman, 1990). This phenomenon appears to occur primarily in adolescents and young adults but not at older ages (Gould et al., 1990). Exposure includes a friend or schoolmate, or even via the media. The effect of media coverage on suicide depends on the amount of coverage, timing of coverage, and duration (Gould, Hendin, & Mann, 2001). Guidelines for safe media coverage of a suicide are available at the Suicide Prevention Resource Center (*www.sprc.org*).

Access to Suicide Attempt Method (Lethal Means)

Statistics suggest that firearms are the most frequent method used by older teenage males who die by suicide in the United States. They are used by 45.4% of males and also by 19.9% of teenage females (ages 15–19 years) who die by suicide (CDC, 2012a). Because many suicide attempts are impulsive in nature, a ready access to a suicide attempt method (particularly a lethal means of suicide, such as a firearm) can heighten risk for suicide. In a pilot

---

Family, Interpersonal, and Contextual Risk Factors

- Family history of psychiatric disorders or suicide
- Physical or sexual abuse
- Bullying, victim of bullying
- Problematic peer relationships, limited social integration
- Poor family support, attachment, communication
- Lesbian, gay, bisexual, or transgender
- Exposure to suicidal behavior
- Access to suicide attempt method

---

study for the National Violent Death Reporting System, evidence suggested that in 82% of the cases in which a firearm was used in a suicide attempt, the firearm belonged to a parent or family member; two-thirds of those firearms were stored unlocked, and in the remaining cases, the youth found the key, or the combination, or broke into the cabinet (Suicide Prevention Resource Center, 2002). Studies are clear that reducing access to lethal means, including firearms, reduces attempts using such means, and may reduce the population suicide rate (Mann et al., 2005).

PROTECTIVE FACTORS FOR TEEN SUICIDE AND SUICIDAL BEHAVIOR

Protective factors are characteristics that are associated with lower levels of suicidal behavior. These factors are often a part of psychological health or well-being, and therefore may protect against suicide as well as a number of other negative health and psychological outcomes. Because the research on protective factors is more limited and because it is difficult to demonstrate that a factor *prevented* something from happening that would have occurred otherwise, there is minimal empirical evidence for protective factors.

Connectedness

Social connectedness may protect against suicidal behavior, suicide, and various associated risk factors (King & Merchant, 2008). Adolescents are affected by support, or the lack thereof, from both family and peers. For instance, as noted above, Lewinsohn et al. (2001) found that low levels of family support were predictive of later suicide attempts for females, whereas low levels of peer support were predictive of suicide attempts for males. Young people who report their families to be supportive and involved are less likely to engage in suicidal behaviors (McKeown et al., 1998; Resnick et al., 1997; Rubenstein, Halton, Kasten, Rubin, & Stechler, 1998; Rubenstein, Heeren, Housman, Rubin, & Stechler, 1989). Moreover, evidence also suggests that social connectedness may enhance adaptive functioning and teen competencies. For example, high levels of support from family are inversely related to adolescents' substance use (Wills & Cleary, 1996), whereas low social support is linked to suicide risk factors, such as depression, conduct problems, and alcohol/substance problems (Kerr, Preuss, & King, 2006; Mazza & Reynolds, 1998; Prinstein, Nock, Spirito, & Grapentine, 2001). Lack of social support is associated with adjustment problems (East, Hess, & Lerner, 1987), social avoidance (La Greca & Lopez, 1998), loneliness (Mahon, Yarcheski, Yarcheski, Cannella, & Hanks, 2006), delinquency, bullying, and both internalizing and externalizing behaviors (Scolte, van Lieshout, & van Aken, 2001). In contrast, social competence and social acceptance are associated with positive interactions (Bierman & McCauley, 1987) and positive adjustment (Peters, 1988).

Good social skills, including decision making and problem solving, also protect against teen suicidal behavior (Jessor, 1991; Rudd et al., 1996). However, studies to support this prediction focus only on improving social skills among those who are at risk. These studies show a decrease in suicidal behavior among these youth (LaFromboise & Howard-Pitney, 1995; Thompson, Eggert, & Herting, 2000; Thompson, Eggert, Randell, & Pike, 2001). As clinicians, we look to these findings when designing crisis response and treatment plans for suicidal teens. We often try to increase support and connections for suicidal teens in their families, schools, and communities and may also work to improve their problem-solving capacities.

CONCLUSION

In this chapter, we have reviewed the demographic, clinical, and family/interpersonal factors that have been empirically shown to convey risk for suicidal behavior among teens, as well as emerging findings about what may protect these teens against that risk. We build on this knowledge base in subsequent chapters as we describe how to screen and formally assess suicidal risk in individual teenagers.

CHAPTER THREE

Screening

How We Recognize Elevated Risk

▶ Review basic principles of screening for suicide risk.

▶ Provide information about evidence-based screening instruments and techniques.

▶ Provide guidelines for suicide risk screening in the following settings:

  ▪ Mental health settings;

  ▪ Medical settings—emergency departments and primary care;

  ▪ Schools.

In the previous chapter, we reviewed the current evidence regarding risk factors for suicidal behavior and suicide among teenagers. Armed with this knowledge, the next step is to identify teens who may be at elevated risk. In this chapter, we review the basic principles of suicide risk screening and provide information about how to develop and implement a screening strategy. We discuss general guidelines for outpatient mental health clinics, emergency departments, and schools. Finally, we share information about commonly used, evidence-based interview and self-report teen suicide risk screening instruments. Tables are provided for easy access to information about these instruments.

Screening involves gathering information to determine whether an individual teen may be at elevated risk for suicidal behavior or suicide. It is the first step in determining whether a comprehensive risk assessment is indicated. In suicide prevention, "screening strategies are based on the valid premise that suicidal adolescents are under-identified, have an active, often treatable mental illness, and exhibit identifiable risk factors" (Gould et al., 2005, p. 1635). This chapter focuses on screening at the individual level. It is acknowledged that screening for prevention may also occur at group and community levels (National Research Council and Institute of Medicine of the National Academies, 2009).

It is important to differentiate a suicide risk screen from a comprehensive suicide risk assessment. *The goal of the suicide risk screen is to cast a wide net to identify teens who may be at elevated risk for suicidal behavior.* As such, these screens are generally brief, may involve only the teen as the informant, and may consist of only a few suicide-related questions. If the screen takes place in a mental health setting, a more comprehensive suicide risk assessment is then conducted with adolescents who screen positive. If the screen takes place in a school setting, adolescents who screen positive are generally referred to a mental health professional for the more comprehensive suicide risk assessment. This assessment is conducted to obtain in-depth information about risk and protective factors, formulate the nature and severity of elevated risk, and determine next steps and a treatment plan (described in Chapter 4).

The clinical and public health potential of suicide risk screening has garnered much national attention in recent years. In fact, screening has been officially recommended as a suicide prevention strategy in a variety of policy documents. For example in 2003, the New Freedom Commission on Mental Health issued a report titled *Achieving the Promise: Transforming Mental Health Care in America* (New Freedom Commission on Mental Health, 2003). This document includes a number of recommendations that support the role of screening in improving the mental health of our nation's youth. These recommendations are consistent with those in earlier policy statements that support screening for specific disorders associated with suicide, including the U.S. Surgeon General's Call to Action to Prevent Suicide (U.S. Public Health Service, 1999) and the National Strategy for Suicide Prevention (U.S. DHHS, 2001). The Garrett Lee Smith Memorial Act, passed in 2004, also strongly supports the implementation of screening strategies and programs in youth-focused settings and institutions. These policy statements converge in their belief that screening for suicide risk factors can benefit youth suicide prevention initiatives at a public health level.

BASIC PRINCIPLES OF SCREENING

Successful screening strategies share three vital characteristics: (1) they are *brief and easy to implement*; (2) they are *evidence based* (reliable and valid); and (3) they *include a plan for communication, documentation, and follow-up*. This chapter provides information for practitioners who work in a variety of settings, including specialized mental health clinics, emergency departments, and schools. In the specialized mental health and emergency settings, the clinicians who screen for suicide risk often also take responsibility for conducting the comprehensive risk assessment and formulation (described in Chapter 4). In schools, screening protocols generally include plans to refer teens who screen positive for suicide risk to a specialized mental health clinic for follow-up and comprehensive risk assessment.

Basic Principles of Suicide Risk Screening

- Brief and easy to implement
- Evidence based (reliable and valid)
- Plan for communication, documentation, and follow-up

Although feasible screening strategies in all settings share these three characteristics, they differ in terms of whether a *self-report questionnaire or interview screen* is used, and in whether an *individualized or group (classroom) screening* approach is taken. In this chapter we discuss each of these types of screening strategies.

It is also possible to differentiate formal screening, which is defined as a proactive, evidence-based screen for elevated suicide risk, from informal screening. *Although formal screening is the primary focus of this chapter, we want to emphasize that informal screening is also important and should be routine practice in all health care, school, and youth-serving agencies.*

Informal screening involves all of us (parents, peers, professionals) "keeping our eyes and ears open" to recognize red flags or signs of possibly elevated risk. Teens who are considering suicide often tell someone of their thoughts, and often this person is a peer (Kalafat & Elias, 1992). Informal sources of information may include a teen's communication with peers verbally or via e-mail, text messaging, or social networking sites such as Facebook or Twitter. Teens may also share their concerns via poetry, song lyrics, short stories, or doodles. At times, teens who are contemplating suicide will make seemingly offhand, subtle comments such as, "It's not going to be a problem anymore," or they may make even more direct comments expressing a wish to die or general thoughts about what it would be like to be dead. These comments may be made to teachers or health care professionals. They may also be made to parents, peers, or others such as the parents of the adolescent's friends. As professionals who work with teens, we can play a role in educating the public about their roles as "gatekeepers," and about the importance of paying attention to these clues and red flags. Informal screening should include asking teens in an empathic, nonjudgmental, but direct fashion about whether they are considering suicide when we become aware of these signs of potential risk. Later on, in Chapter 4 and **Appendix D, Questions to Ask about Suicidal Thoughts**, we provide you with guidance and suggestions for asking such questions.

Brief and Easy to Implement

A successful formal screening procedure must be brief and easily incorporated into routine procedures in an outpatient clinic, emergency medical setting, or school. Despite the importance of finding and intervening with the teen at elevated risk for suicide, it is also important to remember that most teens are not at elevated risk. Moreover, because in some settings we may be screening for "high risk" in multiple domains, such as dating violence, alcohol and drug use, and sexual promiscuity, it is not always feasible to use all available time and resources to screen for suicide risk. To ensure high feasibility of use, screening procedures ideally require only a few additional minutes to implement and do not add substantially to the already extensive workload of mental health and school professionals.

One critical determinant of the success of the suicide screening strategy, then, is the choice of screen interview questions and/or instrument(s). In addition to being evidence-based (discussed below), the chosen instrument should be easy to administer and interpret. If an interview instrument is used, it is best if it is familiar to the mental health professional or school-based counselor, who may need practice or desensitization in asking screen questions about suicide. In the case of a self-report questionnaire, it should be relatively simple and straightforward so that teens with varying reading levels can respond meaningfully.

Evidence Based (Strong Psychometric Properties)

Screening questions and instruments must be psychometrically sound. Table 3.1 describes the key psychometric properties of suicide risk screens. A *reliable* instrument is one that measures a construct (in this case, indicators of suicide risk) consistently across interviewers (interrater reliability), across items (internal consistency), and over time (test–retest reliability). Consistency over time is important only to the extent that the actual level of suicide risk remains the same. A *valid* instrument is one that measures what it purports to measure. Face validity means that the questions

TABLE 3.1. Psychometric Properties of Screens

Reliability

Screen findings are consistent.
- Across interviewers
- Across screen items

Validity

Screen findings capture information that is meaningful to risk for suicidal behavior and suicide.

Sensitivity

Teens at risk for suicidal behavior and suicide screen positive.

Specificity

Teens not at risk for suicidal behavior and suicide do not screen positive.

look like they measure something important to suicide risk. Concurrent validity means that a teen's screen "results" are meaningfully related to "results" from other, perhaps more extensive and already validated measures or interviews pertinent to suicide risk. The predictive validity of a screen refers to its ability to predict suicide-related outcomes, including suicide attempts and death by suicide. If strong, these psychometric characteristics enable us to interpret screen findings in a meaningful way. A positive screen does, indeed, mean that the teen is at elevated risk.

Two other psychometric characteristics that are useful to consider include *sensitivity* and *specificity*. A highly sensitive instrument will correctly identify almost all of the teens who are indeed at increased risk for suicidal behavior or suicide. The higher the level of sensitivity, the less likely it is that our screening instrument will fail to identify a teen who really is at risk. On the other hand, an instrument with strong specificity will refrain from identifying a teen as suicidal who is not at elevated risk.

An instrument's sensitivity and specificity have several important implications, both in terms of feasibility and ethical/legal obligations. A test that is sensitive but not specific will have a high number of false positives. For example, a screening instrument that yields a positive screen for all teens who report depressive symptoms *or* alcohol misuse *or* morbid thoughts would likely identify many—perhaps too many—teens as being at elevated risk. This feature may make screening with such an instrument less feasible, as it would require significantly more time to follow up with all of the teens who would score in the elevated range. On the other hand, one could argue that such an instrument may be preferable, because in the context of suicide prevention efforts, it may be ethically and legally preferable to "cast a wide net" and value false positives over the possibility of missing a teenager who is at real risk of self-harm. Weighing the issues of sensitivity versus specificity is a decision that your setting must make in the context of available resources and priorities.

Plan for Communication, Documentation, and Follow-Up

Prior to embarking on a screening protocol, it is important for a key administrator in your setting to develop a comprehensive communication, documentation, and follow-up policy. Ideally, this will be developed in accordance with the recommendations of experts in risk management and medical documentation (Baerger, 2001). Timely follow-up with each teen who screens positive is vital. When we screen for risk of suicidal behavior, we are obligated to share positive screen information with other important individuals who are responsible for the teenager. This group would include parents and could also include other members of the medical or mental health treatment team, school professionals, and others, depending on the context in which screening is conducted.

If screening occurs in an emergency department, primary care, or school setting, teens may be referred elsewhere for a comprehensive risk assessment and treatment. Before beginning any screening program, your agency should have a clear protocol that guides staff regarding how to facilitate the referral of teens and the steps that are needed to follow up and ensure that the at-risk teen has reached the next level of services. For ethical and risk management purposes, it is recommended that schools, primary care, and emergency settings develop some type of tracking log or template to document the following: (1) name of student who screened positive; (2) when/

whether on-site follow-up was conducted; (3) notification of parents or other professionals, if warranted; (4) recommendations made for services (e.g., mental health treatment/evaluation, substance use treatment, immediate ER evaluation); and (5) follow-up contact to assess utilization of services (did the family make the appointment, was the appointment kept). A partially completed sample of **Appendix B, Tracking Form for School-Based Screening**, appears below:

Student name	Date of positive screen	Date of follow-up	Date parents notified	Referral/ recommendation	Date of follow-up to assess service utilization
Jane Doe	10/1/12	10/1/12 by community psychologist assisting with screening	10/1/12 by Mrs. Smith, school social worker	Comprehensive mental health and substance use evaluation	10/5/12 by Mrs. Smith. Parents report appointment scheduled.

This tracking form must be kept in a confidential and secure location. If the screening takes place in a mental health setting where it is possible to conduct a comprehensive risk assessment, this risk assessment may take place immediately. This is frequently the case when the screen is conducted as one part of an intake evaluation that may include a full diagnostic interview with many probes or screens (e.g., for eating disorders, substance use, sexual abuse). The positive screen for suicide risk is the indicator that a comprehensive suicide risk assessment is indicated. It is also possible, however, that the positive screen results in referral for follow-up with a clinician who has more expertise in suicide risk assessment or more time available for the comprehensive risk assessment. In these instances, the transfer to the other clinician should be communicated and documented, with appropriate follow-up.

When screening takes place in a primary care or emergency department setting, the information obtained could easily be included within a medical record. If the suicide risk screen is positive, communication and follow-up with a comprehensive risk assessment is recommended before the adolescent leaves the setting. In a school setting, the positive screen information often resides with a designated school mental health professional responsible for case management/follow-up services.

Recently, the Substance Abuse and Mental Health Services Administration convened a Lessons Learned Working Group (LLWG) composed of participants from multiple public and private stakeholders (e.g., Suicide Prevention Resource Center, Centers for Disease Control and Prevention, American Foundation for Suicide Prevention), as well as experts in youth suicide screening and those implementing screening programs across the United States with funding from the Garrett Lee Smith Memorial Act. The LLWG has drafted a series of recommendations for agencies considering adopting a youth suicide screening program. These guidelines can be found at the Suicide Prevention Resource Center (*www.sprc. org*; 2012)

In summary, when designing an evidence-based screening strategy, we encourage you to consider the following factors: (1) brevity and feasibility of administration; (2) evidence base, including psychometric strength of the screening instrument; and (3) development of a plan for communication, documentation, and follow-up (including referral if appropriate) that fits with the ethical and legal responsibilities of your profession and setting.

INTERVIEW AND SELF-REPORT SCREENING STRATEGIES

Interview

Most suicide risk screens in mental health settings are conducted face to face, using an interview format. In conducting such an interview, it is important to keep in mind that *one question is insufficient as a suicide risk screen*. A teen may respond "Not really" to a question such as "Have you had any thoughts of suicide?" yet later explain in detail a previous suicidal plan. *We recommend that a suicide risk screen include at least three questions and that questions address, at minimum, current suicidal thoughts and a lifetime history of suicide attempts.* Our interest is in determining whether we need to conduct a comprehensive risk assessment and possibly intervene to lessen the emotional pain and risk for suicide attempt and suicide.

Why the multiquestion approach with a focus on suicidal ideation and history of suicide attempts? In a large, community-based study, Lewinsohn and his colleagues (1996) found that 16.7% of adolescents with high levels of suicidal ideation at baseline made a suicide attempt some time during the year. Other studies converge in finding that 10–18% of adolescents who are hospitalized because of a suicide attempt or acute suicide risk make repeat attempts within the 6 months following their hospitalization (Brent, Kolko, et al., 1993; King, Hovey, Brand, & Wilson, 1997). A prior suicide attempt increases the likelihood of a future suicide attempt, and 30–50% of adolescents who die by suicide have previously attempted suicide (Marttunen, Aro, & Lonnqvist, 1992; Shaffer, 1996). Thus, it is important to ascertain the severity of suicidal ideation and the teen's history of suicide attempts.

The Columbia Suicide Severity Rating Scale (C-SSRS) is a semistructured clinical interview that assesses the types and severity of suicidal ideation and behavior (Posner et al., 2011; Posner, Oquendo, Gould, Stanley, & Davies, 2007). It carefully differentiates and provides clear definitions for actual suicide attempt, interrupted suicide attempt, aborted suicide attempt, and preparatory acts toward making a suicide attempt. Ongoing research will provide information about the extent to which these differing

---

Interview Screen for Elevated Suicide Risk

Do	Do NOT
• Screen early in session/ interview.	• Screen just before patient is leaving your office.
• Maintain calm, collaborative stance.	• Overreact to mention of suicidal thought or impulse.
• Ask directly about suicide thoughts and history of suicide attempts.	• Avoid all references to suicide.
• Use multiple questions.	• Ask only one question.

categories will inform risk formulations and clinical decision making. In addition to these categories of behavior, the C-SSRS includes ratings of the severity (from wish to be dead to suicidal intent with a planned method) and intensity (frequency, duration, controllability, deterrents, reasons). Research has indicated that the C-SSRS has favorable psychometric properties with adolescents, including convergent and predictive validity (King, Gipson, Agarwala, & Opperman, 2011; Posner et al., 2011).

Okay to Ask about Suicide

The issues of safety and "bedside manner" are worthy of some attention. A concern often voiced in the community, and by a small but significant number of mental health professionals, is that asking questions about suicidal thoughts and suicide attempts may somehow "put the idea" in teens' minds or lead to rumination about the possibility of suicide. Fortunately, we have evidence to dispute this. Gould and colleagues conducted an empirical study to examine the impact of responding to questions about suicide on the students' suicidal thoughts and found no negative impact on the students (Gould et al., 2005). If suicide risk screening is conducted in a sensitive and therapeutic manner, there is no reason to believe that it will have a negative impact. Rather, screening questions offer the teen an opportunity and safe context in which to share thoughts he or she may have been struggling with for some time.

How to Ask about Suicide

We have limited empirical evidence to guide us in determining the most effective way to ask questions about suicide. What is the most sensitive way to ask questions about suicide ideation and history of suicide attempt, and, of equal or greater importance, which approach yields the most valid responses? As we await further studies on this, we can go forward and ask these questions using skills that have been associated with the establishment of good therapy alliances and teen disclosures of potentially important yet upsetting information (Karver, Handelsman, Fields, & Bickman, 2006).

CLINICAL NOTE

Questions can be stated in a manner such as, "I'm concerned about you. I'm wondering whether you've ever had thoughts of ending your life (or killing yourself, or suicide)?" Or "Given all of the pain you're in right now and your recent disappointments in school, I'm wondering whether you've ever considered suicide?"

The key is to ask. Questions can be stated in a manner such as, "I'm concerned about you. I'm wondering whether you've ever had thoughts of ending your life (or killing yourself, or suicide)?" Or, "Given all of the pain you're in right now and your recent disappointments in school, I'm wondering whether you've ever considered suicide?" The latter is an example of "shame attenuation," a phrase coined by Shawn Shea, who has written extensively on interviewing suicidal clients (Shea, 1998a, 1998b). By beginning with an empathic statement about the teen's struggles, the question is presented in a sensitive manner and within the context of the teen's current struggles. Shea also describes "normalization," which would be asking the screening questions in a manner such as, "Many teens, when they are struggling with a clinical depression and have experienced a trauma like this, experience thoughts of suicide. I'm wondering if you've had any thoughts about suicide." This phrasing suggests that the teen is not alone in his or her struggles or in having suicidal thoughts. It also suggests that the clinician has some experience in dealing with suicidal teens.

Most commonly used suicide screening and risk assessment tools begin with a somewhat general question about thoughts of death. Although we do not have empirical evidence concerning the most effective sequence of questions (in terms of identifying valid cases of suicide risk), this strategy flows well clinically and is generally thought to desensitize the teenager to a sensitive area of inquiry.

Table 3.2 provides information about commonly used interviews for teen suicidal ideation and behavior. It lists the sequence of questions used in major diagnostic instruments for children and adolescents, which begin with a question about morbid thoughts.

TABLE 3.2. Commonly Used Interviews for Assessing Teen Suicidal Ideation and Behavior

Instrument	Sample questions
The Schedule for Affective Disorders and Schizophrenia for School-Age Children: Present and Lifetime Version (KSADS-PL; Kaufman et al., 1997)	Sometimes children who get upset or feel bad wish they were dead or feel they'd be better off dead. Have you ever had these types of thoughts? When? Do you feel that way now? Was there ever another time you felt that way?
	Sometimes children who get upset or feel bad think about dying or even killing themselves. Have you ever had such thoughts? How would you do it? Did you have a plan?
Columbia Suicide Severity Rating Scale (C-SSRS, Posner et al., 2009)	Have you wished you were dead or wished you could go to sleep and not wake up?
	Have you actually had any thoughts of killing yourself?
	Have you been thinking about how you might do this?
	Have you had these thoughts and had some intention of acting on them?
	Have you started to work out or worked out the details of how to kill yourself? Do you intend to carry out this plan?
Diagnostic Interview Schedule for Children (Youth Informant) (DISC-IV; Shaffer et al., 2004)	In the last year [or alternate time period], was there a time when you often thought about death or about people who had died or about being dead yourself? [This is followed by specific questions.]
	In the last year [or alternate time period], was there a time when you thought seriously about killing yourself?
	a. Did you think about killing yourself many times in the last year?
	b. In the last year, did you have a plan for exactly how you would kill yourself?
	c. Did you think a lot about suicide during the time you felt [sad or depressed/like nothing was fun/grouchy]?
Children's Interview for Psychiatric Syndromes (ChIPS; Rooney, Fristad, Weller, & Weller, 1999)	When you feel [_____],
	a. Do you ever wish you were dead?
	b. Do you ever think life isn't worth living?
	c. Have you ever thought of suicide [killing yourself]? If yes, ask:
	d. Have you ever thought about how you would hurt yourself? If yes: What would you do?
	e. Have you ever tried to kill yourself?

One example from the C-SSRS (Posner et al., 2008) is as follows: "Have you wished you were dead or wished you could go to sleep and not wake up?" Similarly, the Diagnostic Interview Schedule for Children (DISC-IV; Shaffer, Fisher, Lucas, Hilsenroth, & Segal, 2004) begins this line of questioning with, "In the last year (or alternate time period) was there a time when you often thought about death or about people who had died or about being dead yourself?" This initial question is then followed by more specific questions regarding thoughts of suicide. For example, the DISC-IV asks, "In the last year (or alternate time period), was there a time when you thought seriously about killing yourself?" The Schedule for Affective Disorders and Schizophrenia for School-Age Children: Present and Lifetime Version (KSADS-PL; Kaufman, Birmaher, Brent, & Rao, 1997) follows its initial question with: "Sometimes children who get upset or feel bad think about dying or even killing themselves. Have you ever had such thoughts?"

Self-Report Screens

Self-report screens may have several advantages as an initial screening strategy in many settings and as an adjunct to the clinical interview in mental health settings. These instruments are often standardized and have known psychometric properties. Furthermore, they require minimal personnel time for administration. Computerized self-report assessment methods may be especially useful in obtaining information about sensitive topics (Hamann, Larkin, Brown, Schwann, & George, 2007; Tourangeau & Yan, 2007; Turner et al., 1998).

Suicidal Ideation Questionnaire—Junior

The Suicidal Ideation Questionnaire—Junior (SIQ-JR; Reynolds, 1988) is an easy-to-read self-report screen that was originally developed for school settings. It has 15 items and can be completed by adolescents in 1 to 3 minutes. The SIQ-JR has demonstrated good internal consistency reliability with a Cronbach's coefficient alpha of .94 for a large standardization sample. It has also demonstrated test–retest reliability (.72) over a 4-week span among a group of high school students, and excellent construct validity, with significant correlations found between the SIQ-JR and measures of depression and hopelessness (Reynolds, 1988). Furthermore, it has shown evidence of predictive validity for suicide thoughts and attempts across a 6-month period following hospitalization (Huth-Bocks, Kerr, Ivey, Kramer, & King, 2007; King, Hovey, Brand, & Ghaziuddin, 1997). Although a longer "high school" version was also developed, the SIQ-JR has been shown to work well with adolescents of all ages.

What are the drawbacks of the SIQ-JR as a screen for elevated risk of suicidal behavior and suicide? Although it requires only 1–3 minutes for completion, it could be argued that 15 items is too long for a screening instrument. In addition, it assesses only suicidal ideation, and research suggests that suicidal ideation is a stronger predictor of subsequent suicidal behavior in girls than in boys (King, Jiang, Czyz, & Kerr, 2012; Lewinsohn et al., 2001). Thus the SIQ-JR has some limitations as a clinical screening tool, particularly for boys.

Beck Scale for Suicide Ideation

The Beck Scale for Suicide Ideation (Beck & Steer, 1991) is a 21-item self-report scale. The first 19 items assess the severity of the individual's suicidal wishes, attitudes, and plans; the last two items assess the number of previous suicide attempts and the level of suicidal intent associated with the most recent suicide attempt (Beck & Steer, 1991). Importantly, this scale gauges plans and preparations for a suicide attempt. It has been used much more in adult rather than adolescent samples. However, this scale was found to have strong psychometric properties and concurrent validity in a study of suicidal ideation among adolescent inpatients (Steer, Kumar, & Beck, 1993a, 1993b). The internal consistency was exceptionally high, and scores correlated positively with adolescents' scores for the Beck Depression Inventory and Beck Hopelessness Scale. They also were associated with a history of a past suicide attempt. Additional research is needed regarding the predictive validity of the Beck Scale for Suicide Ideation for boys and girls.

Youth Risk Behavior Survey

The Youth Risk Behavior Survey (YRBS; CDC, 2011) is a national survey that has been conducted many times to examine the prevalence of a wide range of youth risk behaviors. The YRBS includes five questions that assess sadness or hopelessness, serious thoughts of suicide, existence of a suicide attempt plan, and actual suicide attempts and their lethality (Figure 3.1). As such, these questions could stand alone as a screen for suicidal thoughts, intent, and behavior. Much of the nationally representative data we have concerning the prevalence of suicidal ideation and behavior among teens comes from the YRBS.

DIRECTIONS: The next five questions ask about sad feelings and attempted suicide. Sometimes people feel so depressed about the future that they may consider attempting suicide, that is, taking some action to end their own life.	
Question	**Answer Choices**
During the past 12 months, did you ever feel so sad or hopeless almost every day for **2 weeks or more in a row** that you stopped doing some usual activities?	Yes, No
During the past 12 months, did you ever **seriously** consider attempting suicide?	Yes, No
During the past 12 months, did you make a plan about how you would attempt suicide?	Yes, No
During the past 12 months, how many times did you actually attempt suicide?	0 times, 1 time, 2 or 3 times, 4 or 5 times, 6 or more times
If you attempted suicide during the past 12 months, did any attempt result in an injury, poisoning, or overdose that had to be treated by a doctor or nurse?	**I did not attempt suicide** during the past 12 months Yes No

FIGURE 3.1. State and Local Youth Risk Behavior Survey: Questions assessing suicide attempts and ideation (CDC, 2011).

Self-Report Surveys Assessing Multiple Risk Factors

Because suicidal ideation and prior suicide attempts are not the only risk factors for teen suicide, some screening strategies assess multiple risk factors. These strategies either entail administration of one comprehensive screening instrument or a combination of brief screening instruments.

The TeenScreen Program makes use of a general health questionnaire with items embedded within it to assess depression, anxiety, substance abuse, and suicidal thoughts and behaviors. Some items have a yes/no response format; other items make use of a 5-point Likert scale. One advantage of the TeenScreen is that it screens for a broader array of known suicide risk factors. As such, it may be a stronger screen for actually elevated suicide risk (more research is needed on this), and it may identify teens at risk for other negative outcomes. In addition, the TeenScreen questionnaire has shown good concurrent validity (Shaffer, Scott, et al., 2004).

Multicomponent screens have also been developed for use with adolescents who present to medical emergency departments. As an example of one of the early approaches in this area, Horowitz and colleagues (2001) developed a screen for children and adolescents who presented to the emergency department with psychiatric chief complaints. In addition to the customary psychiatric evaluation, patient participants completed a screening survey that included a 14-item Risk of Suicide Questionnaire (RSQ) and the 30-item Suicidal Ideation Questionnaire (SIQ). The RSQ assessed suicidal thoughts and behaviors, life stress, alcohol and drug use, and interpersonal loss. They found that four of the RSQ items were most predictive of their criterion standard (i.e., SIQ scores). In the realm of screening instruments, this combination of scales is relatively long. Although the RSQ is promising, data are not available regarding how scores on this screen relate to suicide attempts or other risk indicators.

In recognition of the potential offered by medical emergency departments as sites for screening large numbers of adolescents at possibly elevated risk, King, O'Mara, Hayward, & Cunningham (2009) developed a suicide risk screen for adolescents who present with either psychiatric or nonpsychiatric chief complaints. Because many of these adolescents present with complaints that would not generally trigger a psychiatric or mental health evaluation—such as accidental injury, alcohol/drug overdose, or exacerbation of chronic medical illness—and because the mission of the medical emergency department is to focus on emergencies and acute conditions, King and colleagues focused on identifying a high-risk group of adolescents. They used a combination of brief screen instruments to assess whether adolescents reported: (1) severe suicidal thoughts and/or recent suicide attempt, and/or (2) co-occurring depression and alcohol/substance abuse (King, O'Mara, et al., 2009). Specifically, they used the SIQ-JR, the Reynolds Adolescent Depression Scale–2: Short Form (RADS-2: SF; Reynolds, 2008) and the three-item Alcohol Use Disorders Identification Test—Consumption (AUDIT-C; Reinert & Allen, 2007). In their examination of the validity and utility of this screening survey, 16% of teens screened positive for suicide risk; 18% of these teens had presented for non-psychiatric reasons. This result suggests the potential of such a screen strategy to identify teens at elevated risk for suicide.

Even more recently, clinical researchers have begun to make use of Web- or Internet-based screening platforms. Fein and colleagues (2010) examined the use of a Web-based screening tool that assesses mental health concerns (e.g. depression, posttraumatic stress), psychosocial concerns (family violence), and suicide risk among teens who are seeking emergency medical services for non-psychiatric complaints (Fein et al., 2010). In an initial evaluation of this approach, which involves emergency services staff conducting and interpreting the screen, approximately 10% of participating teens screened positive and were further evaluated. Similarly, Diamond and colleagues developed a Behavioral Health Screen (BHS) for adolescents and young adults, ages 12–21 years, seeking primary care services (Diamond et al., 2010). They documented an administration time of 8–15 minutes (54 items with up to 39 follow-up items) and acceptable to strong psychometric properties, particularly in terms of predicting risk behaviors.

These studies each have promising findings and highlight the possibility of screening for elevated suicide risk using a combination of brief screening instruments or items that tap multiple suicide risk factors.

Comparison of Interview and Self-Report Screen Strategies

Taken together, there are several options for screening strategies. These include a self-report questionnaire that specifically assesses suicidal thoughts and requires only a few minutes to administer (SIQ-JR), a series of questions that take a broader look at a wide spectrum of suicidal thoughts and behaviors (C-SSRS, YRBS), a combination of brief screen instruments that tap suicidal thoughts and behaviors in addition to depression and alcohol/substance abuse (Diamond et al., 2010; Fein et al., 2010; King, O'Mara, et al., 2009) or a general health questionnaire such as TeenScreen. Comparative data are unavailable to clearly guide your decision regarding which screen instrument to use. If larger numbers of teens are to be screened who do not present specifically with suicidal concerns or psychiatric complaints, and if time is limited in the setting, a self-report method may be preferable. If trained mental health professionals are available in the setting, an interview approach or an interview combined with a brief screen may be preferable.

SCREENING STRATEGIES FOR YOUR SETTING

Mental Health Settings

It is recommended that all teens evaluated or treated in any type of mental health setting be screened for elevated suicide risk. This recommendation is consistent with the practice guidelines of mental health professions (e.g., American Academy of Child and Adolescent Psychiatry, 2001). This screening should take place early in the session or interview so there is sufficient time to conduct a comprehensive risk assessment if there are any signs of possibly elevated risk. In the outpatient or inpatient mental health setting, this screen is almost always conducted in person as part of a clinical interview. It may be useful, however, to supplement this interview screen with a self-report screen, particularly given research indicating that teens may be more likely to share potentially stigmatizing concerns via self-report rather than when they are face to face with an adult in an office setting (Klimes-Dougan, 1998; Safer, 1997).

When conducting the interview screen and when sharing findings from the self-report screen, it is important for the clinician to maintain a calm, nonjudgmental manner—accepting the teen's responses without overreacting with shock, a statement like "but you have so much going for you," or a knee-jerk reaction to immediately arrange psychiatric hospitalization. The goal is to elicit the most valid or honest information possible from the teen, and to understand his or her psychological pain and the problems that are driving it. Additional information about interviewing strategies commonly used in mental health settings is presented above, in the section on interview screens. Finally, Chapter Four presents substantial information about the comprehensive suicide risk assessment and formulation, which are generally conducted in the mental health setting.

Medical Settings: Emergency Departments and Primary Care Clinics

Medical settings offer multiple advantages for suicide risk screening. First, most young people visit a primary care provider at least once each year (as reviewed in Tylee, Haller, Graham, Churchill, & Sanci, 2007), and approximately 30% of adolescents seek medical emergency services each year (Britto, Klostermann, Bonny, Altum, & Hornung, 2001). Given that many adolescents have limited knowledge concerning available mental health services (Fotheringham & Sawyer, 1995) and just over one-third (36%) of adolescents with mental disorders get professional help, as reported in a nationally representative sample of 6,483 adolescents (Merikangas et al., 2011), proactive screening and follow-up may be necessary to reach more adolescents and engage them in treatment.

This need for proactive screening may be particularly acute for identifiable subgroups of adolescents. It is well established that mental health service utilization varies by gender, minority status, and age. Adolescent girls are more likely than adolescent boys to receive treatment for anxiety disorders, whereas adolescent boys are more likely than adolescent girls to receive treatment for attention-deficit/hyperactivity disorder (Merikangas et al., 2011). Adolescents who are racial/ethnic minorities (Hispanic and non-Hispanic Black) are less likely to receive treatment for mood and anxiety disorders than white adolescents, even when these conditions are associated with substantial functional impairment (Merikangas et al., 2011). There are also differences across childhood and adolescence in mental health service use patterns (Cuffe et al., 2001). Young adolescents with significant mental health concerns are more likely to have contact with mental health professionals than middle adolescents who, in turn, are more likely to have contact with mental health professionals than older adolescents. Finally, older adolescent boys account for a lower percentage of total health care visits than younger adolescent boys, despite increases in girls' health care use during this same time frame (Marcell & Halpern-Felsher, 2005).

Given these data on limited and variable mental health service use among adolescents, it is not surprising that most adolescents who die by suicide have never received any type of psychiatric treatment or mental health service (Brent et al., 1988; Marttunen et al., 1992; Shaffer et al., 1996). The decline in mental health service use among older versus younger teens, and particularly among older males, is particularly disconcerting given the higher suicide rate among boys and the rise in the suicide rate from early to late adolescence.

Screening in the Emergency Department

The emergency department has several advantages as a screening site. First, large numbers of adolescents seek emergency services each year, and some of these adolescents obtain both routine and emergency health care in these settings (Wilson & Klein, 2000). Second, the significant wait times common in emergency settings may offer an opportunity to screen adolescents without creating the burden of an additional time requirement. Third, the emergency department offers an opportunity to screen a broad sample of adolescents from the community, including those who present with conditions associated with elevated suicide risk such as alcohol poisoning, auto accident injury, suicide attempt, bullying victimization, and intentional injury from a violent altercation.

Screening strategies in emergency departments need to place a strong emphasis on feasibility, as these settings are extremely busy and often overburdened. In keeping with the recommendations at the beginning of this chapter, these strategies must be brief, easily understood by patients, and readily administered and interpreted in busy general hospital settings. Nevertheless, several recent studies suggest that such screening is feasible for adolescent patients who present with psychiatric and nonpsychiatric chief complaints (Fein et al., 2010; Horowitz et al., 2010; King, O'Mara, et al., 2009).

There are a number of screening instruments and strategies that could be used, abbreviated and/or adapted for use in emergency departments. Several of these were described earlier in this chapter, including the Columbia Suicide Severity Rating Scale (C-SSRS; Posner et al., 2008), the Suicidal Ideation Questionnaire–Junior (SIQ-JR; Reynolds, 1988), and several multifactor screening tools (Fein et al., 2010; Horowitz et al., 2010; King, O'Mara, et al., 2009; Wintersteen, Diamond, & Fein, 2007). Issues to be considered include: (1) the number of questions about suicide that minimally but optimally screen for suicide risk; (2) the method of screening that best elicits valid responses to screening questions (and is feasible, acceptable to staff and patients, and cost effective); and (3) the ways in which the results of suicide screening may optimally be conveyed to physicians so that appropriate care is provided to address suicide risk. These issues line up with the three principles of suicide risk screening described at the beginning of this chapter.

In the emergency department, as in outpatient clinics and schools, suicide screening questions may be embedded within broader assessments of mental health and high-risk behaviors (Claassen & Larkin, 2005; Lowenstein et al., 1998; Rhodes et al.,

2001) or asked independently (Folse, Eich, Hall, & Ruppman, 2006; King, O'Mara, et al., 2009 ; Wintersteen et al., 2007). The decision regarding which instrument or combination of instruments to use will likely depend on what can most easily be incorporated into existing procedures while still yielding accurate and useful results.

Fortunately, although we must be cautious in assuming that all adolescents will respond in valid ways to self-report screens (King et al., 2012), recent research indicates that most adolescents and parents have favorable attitudes toward suicide risk screening in the emergency department (Horowitz et al., 2010; O'Mara, Hill, Cunningham, & King, 2012). Adolescents and parents do, however, express concerns related to privacy (O'Mara et al., 2012; Pailler et al., 2009) and the time required for the screening (O'Mara et al., 2012). In a survey of health care providers regarding their beliefs about adolescent depression screening in the emergency department, they expressed concerns about the availability of timely and appropriate follow-up for those adolescents who screen positive (Cronholm et al., 2010). This emphasizes one of the basic principles of suicide risk screening: the importance of a plan for communication, documentation, and follow-up. There must be someone available to speak with the adolescent who screens positive and to follow up as appropriate. The screening protocol and infrastructure for documentation and follow-up requires administrative support within the emergency department.

Screening in Primary Care Settings

The primary care medical setting also offers an opportunity for early detection of elevated suicide risk. A number of medical and mental health professional groups as well as government and policy organizations support screening and early identification for mental health and suicide risk in primary care settings (American Academy of Child and Adolescent Psychiatry, 2009; National Research Council and Institute of Medicine of the National Academies, 2009; New Freedom Commission on Mental Health, 2003; U.S. DHHS, 2001).

More than 70% of adolescents visit their primary care provider at least once a year (Frankenfield et al., 2000), and psychological autopsy studies suggest that 45–66% of individuals who died by suicide had seen their primary care provider in the month prior to their death (Luoma et al., 2002). Despite this finding, only 23% of pediatricians and family practice physicians report that they routinely survey their patients about suicide risk factors (Frankenfield et al., 2000). In another survey regarding adolescent patients, depression was reported as a diagnosis in only 2–3% of primary care outpatient visits (Frankenfield et al., 2000).

A recent study suggests that a standardized primary care screening program to assess suicide risk in adolescents is effective in increasing rates of inquiry, case detection, and referral (Wintersteen, 2010). This screen strategy embedded two standardized questions within the semistructured psychosocial interview portion of the electronic medical chart. Taking advantage of the electronic medical chart format, these questions were automatically included in the interview for adolescents between the ages of 12 and 18 years. The screening implementation program involved a 90-minute training for physicians. The questions assessed morbid ideation ("Have you ever felt that life is not worth living?") and suicidal ideation ("Have you ever felt like you wanted to kill yourself?"). The inclusion of these two questions on the standardized interview increased rates of inquiry by 219% and case detection by 392%, with all at-risk youth referred for mental health follow-up. This study did not follow youth over time and therefore does not include data on outcomes as a result of screening.

Taking a different approach, the same team of investigators have developed a behavioral health screen (BHS) for adolescents and young adults seeking primary care services. Rather than relying on the physician's semistructured interview regarding psychosocial and mental health issues, this is an Internet-based self-report screening strategy. As noted earlier in this chapter, these clinical researchers have reported promising initial findings for this strategy, and their research is ongoing.

Taken together, a number of readily available screening tools may be feasible for use within the primary care setting. Options for both interview and self-report screens were described earlier in this chapter. The primary barriers to implementing mental health and suicide screening in pediatric primary care are physician time, perceptions of inadequate training, ambiguity about whether mental health screening is a responsibility of primary care providers, and reimbursement (Olson et al., 2002). The TeenScreen Primary Care project has recently released a guide for primary care physicians regarding effective reimbursement strategies for mental health screening and follow-up (TeenScreen Primary Care, 2012). There has also been a white paper recently released by SAMHSA titled "Reimbursement of Mental Health Services in Primary Care Settings" (Kautz, Mauch, & Smith, 2008).

As noted by Sanci, Lewis, and Patton (2010), evidence is very limited for the effectiveness of primary care screening in reducing the overall burden of emotional disorders such as depression. There is concern about the possible harm associated with false positives, including enhanced stigma and a strain on already limited health care resources. There are also issues regarding the availability of appropriate treatments and services, and about the adolescent's readiness to use these services. Sanci and colleagues suggest that for screening to be effective in primary care settings, it may need to involve "facilitated" access to effective treatment options, perhaps within a collaborative model of care, for those who screen positive. This issue of access to services is pertinent to all screening settings, including medical emergency departments and schools, as discussed next.

School Settings

Our nation's schools are the most natural place to reach large numbers of adolescents; more than 52 million youth attend more than 114,000 schools in the United States (New Freedom Commission on Mental Health, 2003). School-based strategies for suicide prevention have traditionally included three types: (1) curriculum-based education/awareness programs, (2) staff inservice trainings, and (3) schoolwide screening approaches (Gould, Greenberg, Velting, & Shaffer, 2003). Curriculum-based programs include mental health education and education about warning signs for suicide. These programs tend to encourage students to seek professional help for themselves and to seek help for their peers, if needed. Inservice training programs offer gatekeeper training to teachers and other school staff related to recognizing and responding to risk factors in students. Schoolwide screening programs offer a universal, preventive approach to detecting at-risk adolescents. In keeping with the focus of this chapter, formal school-based screening programs are described below.

A universal approach to suicide prevention is one in which every student in a certain grade or within the school building is screened, as opposed to limiting screening to students who meet some elevated risk criteria. This type of public health approach to suicide prevention is similar to universal prevention strategies such as school-based hearing and vision screening for youth or universally applied substance abuse or pregnancy prevention programs. In addition to the possibility of reaching every student within a school, universal screening programs also have the potential to detect youth who are at elevated but not severe risk. Early detection of subthreshold levels of risk may enable them to avoid a worsening of their illness via early intervention, thereby preventing future suicidal ideation and behavior. Given statistics suggesting that a majority of adolescents who die by suicide have never been seen by a mental health professional (Brent et al., 1988; Marttunen et al., 1992), some type of outreach initiative that facilitates contact with potentially at-risk adolescents is critical.

Available evidence suggests that universal, schoolwide screening programs (1) identify youth who are at elevated risk for suicide (e.g., Pena & Caine, 2006); (2) identify youth who are not currently receiving psychiatric treatments (e.g., Garlow et al., 2008; Scott et al., 2008); and (3) may increase the likelihood that these youth will receive treatment (Gould et al., 2009). Only two studies to date, however, have demonstrated a significant reduction in suicide attempts as a function of widespread school-based screening (Aseltine & DeMartino, 2004, but see discussion below for caveats; Rotheram-Borus & Bradley, 1991). Clearly, much more research is needed to investigate this relatively new area for suicide prevention and intervention.

Below, we present brief information on two well-established, evidence-based schoolwide screening programs, the TeenScreen Program and the (SOS) Signs of Suicide Prevention Program. Both are listed on the National Registry of Evidence-Based Programs and Practices. They are also referenced in **Appendix C, Suicide Prevention Resources for Schools (Guidelines and Education/ Awareness Programs).**

TeenScreen Program

The overall objective of the TeenScreen program has been to provide teens with a free voluntary mental health check-up during their school year. Although the TeenScreen program is currently in transition, we have learned much from it over the years and, in many ways, it serves as a model program. This program has required both parental consent and student assent prior to participation. Students have then completed a 10-minute self-report questionnaire that assesses depression, anxiety, substance abuse, and suicidal thoughts and behaviors. If the teen's responses suggest areas of concern, he or she is referred to a second stage of evaluation with a trained mental health professional located on site. If, at this stage, the mental health professional recommends a more extensive evaluation or treatment, parents are notified and an appropriate referral is made. Studies suggest that the TeenScreen Program successfully identifies students at risk for suicide and increases service utilization (Husky, McGuire, Flynn, Chrostowski, & Olfson, 2009; Scott et al., 2008; Shaffer, Scott, et al., 2004), although more research is needed and forthcoming about this program.

Signs of Suicide Prevention Program

Signs of Suicide (SOS; *www.mentalhealthscreening.org/highschool*) incorporates a curriculum-based classroom intervention (video and discussion guide) with a brief, self-administered self-screening questionnaire aimed at improving self-recognition of depression and suicide risk among students. The program's goals are to teach teens how to recognize the signs of distress in themselves or a friend and respond effectively using the ACT® approach (acknowledge, care, and tell). Students also receive community resources for treatment. SOS does not follow the two-phase model of screening, in which a positive screen results in an immediate evaluation by a mental health professional. Rather, the SOS screen is self-administered and self-scored, and students are encouraged to seek their own treatment if they score in an elevated range. In a randomized controlled trial of the SOS program, Aseltine and DeMartino (2004) found a significant reduction in suicide attempts (by 40%) but no increase in help-seeking for youths 3 months after completing the SOS program compared to youth who received a typical health/social studies class. Other studies (Aseltine, James, Schilling, & Glanovsky, 2007) have replicated the reduction in suicide attempts and have also demonstrated benefits in help seeking (Aseltine, 2003). Although it is one of the few studies to demonstrate an impact on suicide attempts, it is unclear whether the effects of SOS are due to the screening component, the education component, or the combination of the two approaches.

Important Considerations

Although many researchers and suicide prevention advocates see value in schoolwide screening approaches, these strategies face a number of barriers to widespread adoption by schools and communities. School personnel cite concerns about false-positive rates, about resources needed to implement screening appropriately, and about ethical/legal concerns regarding linking students to services (Eckert, Miller, DuPaul, & Riley-Tillman, 2003; Eckert, Miller, Riley-Tillman, & DuPaul, 2006; Scherff, Eckert, & Miller, 2005). In addition to considering the resources needed to conduct follow-up interviews of students with elevated risk scores, lack of available and competent community providers, long wait lists, and lack of adequate mental health insurance, are all ethical and legal concerns that must be addressed in order for a screening program to be implemented safely and effectively. Politically, schoolwide screening also has been controversial, as many see it as intrusive and an invasion of privacy.

Figure 3.2 is a checklist of issues to consider and resolve if your school or community is interested in establishing a formal screening program. These issues are also applicable to primary care or other youth-serving agencies, such as foster care or juvenile justice settings.

CONCLUSION

Suicide risk screening strategies that are relatively brief, feasible, and psychometrically sound are available for use with adolescents in mental health, primary care, emergency department, and school settings. In this chapter, we reviewed basic principles of suicide risk screening (brevity, ease of administration, psychometric

---

1. Assess staff and community resources. Who is trained and available to help both inside (school mental health professionals) and outside (local mental health providers, universities, other community agencies) the school or agency?

2. Form a planning committee with all stakeholders: parents, youth, educators, primary care and mental health professionals, other agencies that include child welfare, juvenile justice, and other relevant child-serving local agencies, and school district legal consultants.

3. Create a memorandum of understanding with community partners to clarify responsibilities. Who will follow up with teens who screen positive? Who will accept referrals?

4. Address logistical details: When during the school day and school year will screening occur? How will follow-ups be handled? How will parental consent be obtained? Where will teens who do not have parental consent go?

5. Who will provide training, supervision, and technical support?

6. How will liability issues be addressed?

FIGURE 3.2. Checklist for implementing a mental health screening program. Based on Weist, Rubin, Moore, Adelsheim, and Wrobel (2007).

quality, and the need to plan for communication, documentation, and follow-up). In addition, we provided information about how to interview teens about their suicidal thoughts, intentions, and behaviors. We also reviewed self-report questionnaires that could be incorporated into a screening program in your setting. Finally, we described strategies for implementing screening procedures in mental health, emergency, school, and primary care settings.

CHAPTER FOUR

Suicide Risk Assessment and Risk Formulation

CHAPTER OBJECTIVES

▶ Review basic principles of risk assessment and formulation.

▶ Describe the steps in risk assessment and formulation.

- Express caring attitude and willingness to help;

- Gather comprehensive information about risk and protective factors;

- Integrate information to formulate risk;

- Document and communicate the risk formulation and plan.

In this chapter, we review the basic principles of risk assessment and formulation, providing practical information that you can use in your professional setting. We provide concrete, easy-to-follow information to guide your risk assessments, including information about the overall approach, the clinical interview, and the use of supplemental self-report questionnaires. A specific inquiry into the adolescent's suicidal thoughts, impulses, history of suicidal behavior, and the mental status exam are emphasized. Finally, we provide guidelines for the process of risk formulation and emphasize the importance of careful documentation. At the conclusion of the chapter, we offer special considerations for clinicians working in an acute care setting and discuss the decision to hospitalize within the context of information gathered during the risk assessment.

A *comprehensive suicide risk assessment* and *risk formulation* are usually completed by licensed mental health professionals. Although there are exceptions, such as physicians and nurses who are trained to complete suicide risk assessments in medical emergency departments, it requires substantial training to do the following: (1) understand the wide array of suicide risk factors and the difference between underlying chronic risk factors (which may be highly significant, yet distal and not acute) and acute risk factors; (2) conduct a sensitive and effective interview to evaluate risk; (3) collect supplementary information using standardized assessment tools as well as interviews with other informants; (4) weigh risk and protective factors to formulate risk; (5) make a clinical judgment about level of risk, with particular attention to acute risk; (6) implement the action plan for the adolescent while, ideally, securing the adolescent's buy-in with the plan; and (7) document this process in a clear manner.

This chapter provides trained mental health professionals with the additional specialized knowledge and tools needed to conduct a suicide risk assessment and formulation. Although all health professionals and many "gatekeepers" such as parents and teachers play an important role in either screening for or recognizing possible suicide risk, individuals with specific mental health expertise are best prepared to conduct the comprehensive suicide risk assessment with potentially suicidal teens. Despite the fact that it is very difficult, perhaps impossible, to predict precisely *who* will make a suicide attempt or die by suicide, and *when* this will occur, a comprehensive risk assessment and formulation provides our best information about whether a teen is at elevated risk for suicidal behavior and suicide and the extent of that risk. This enables appropriate steps to be taken to maintain the teen's safety, promote positive coping, and address risk factors with available evidence-based treatments.

BASIC PRINCIPLES OF RISK ASSESSMENT

There are four basic principles of risk assessment. The first is that *risk can be understood*. Substantial research, conducted over more than 25 years, has provided us with rich information about risk and protective factors for suicidal behavior and suicide among teens. The findings from these studies converge. Many of the same risk factors show up again and again, regardless of whether the study is conducted in an acute psychiatric inpatient setting, an outpatient clinic, or a community setting. As examples, we now have dozens of studies pointing to the importance of risk factors such as a previous suicide attempt, clinical depression, and alcohol abuse. It is our responsibility to know these risk factors and the risk factors unique to the individual teen so that we can conduct a thorough assessment. (Please see Chapter 2 for a full review of risk and protective factors for adolescent suicidal behavior and suicide.) It is also important that we understand that risk is usually multifaceted. Because of this, a comprehensive risk assessment requires the evaluation of multiple potential risk factors as well as an understanding of how these factors may interact with one another.

Principles of Risk Assessment

- Risk can be understood. It requires the assessment of multiple factors.
- Risk is not static. Therefore, assessment must be ongoing.
- Risk does not always "shout out." Therefore, a focused, specific assessment of suicidal thoughts and impulses is recommended.
- Multiple informants facilitate a comprehensive risk assessment.

The second principle of risk assessment is that *risk is not static and therefore assessment must be ongoing.* In Chapter 2 we discussed *chronic versus acute risk factors,* a distinction that is critical to ongoing assessment. In mental health settings, many if not most of our teen clients or patients have one or more chronic risk factors for suicide. These risk factors may include a previous suicide attempt; chronic depressive, bipolar, or other psychiatric disorder; a history of physical abuse, sexual abuse, or other form of victimization; or a family history of suicide in a parent. Epidemiological research indicates that teens with these characteristics or life histories are, as a group, at elevated risk for suicidal behavior and suicide. The exact degree of elevated risk for an individual teen is difficult to estimate. Partially because of this, it is important to monitor these teens closely and assess their level of acute risk at regular intervals. A clinically depressed teen with a history of a suicide attempt may be at high acute risk when under the influence of alcohol or following a disciplinary action or relationship breakup. Before we can formulate risk, we must understand the teen's chronic underlying risk factors and gather as much information as possible to guide our judgment about the teen's level of acute risk.

The third principle of risk assessment is that *risk does not always shout out.* This may be the most challenging aspect of assessing teen suicide risk for mental health professionals, and it is a painful aspect of suicide risk for clinician and family survivors of a suicide. Knowledge of suicide risk factors and repeated suicide risk assessments (with careful risk formulations) are extremely important to preventing suicidal behavior and suicide among teens. Some teens, however, choose not to share information about their suicidal thoughts, impulses, and plans with a parent or mental health professional. This could be for many possible reasons: perhaps because they fear others' strong emotional or negative reactions, or because they can't find the words or courage to share their thoughts, or because they have been to the emergency department or inpatient unit before and do not want to return, or perhaps because they do not want someone to abort or interrupt their plan to die by suicide. Because of this, we recommend a specific inquiry about suicidal thoughts, impulses, and behaviors (described on page 79), a *multi-informant strategy* (described next), and *multiple methods of assessment* (interview, observation, standardized assessment instrument).

The fourth principle of risk assessment is that *multiple informants facilitate a comprehensive assessment.* Depending on the setting and interpersonal context, the adolescent may not reveal all important information, such as information about past suicide attempts, histories of alcohol abuse or conduct disorder, or a previous hospitalization in another setting. Moreover, the adolescent may not have detailed information about previous clinical providers. In these instances, the parent or other legal guardian is frequently able to provide some of the missing information. Furthermore, even when the adolescent is willing and able to share much essential information, the parent, teacher, counselor, and previous providers can provide supplemental information and another perspective on the teen's level of functioning and suicide risk.

We must use caution when interpreting discrepancies among informants. In general, evidence suggests that parents may have limited knowledge about the extent of their adolescent's suicidal ideation or even previous attempts (Klaus, Mobilio, & King, 2009). This is in contrast to findings from several studies focusing on adults (DeJong & Overholser, 2009; Li & Phillips, 2008), which suggest a relatively high degree of concordance between the reports of suicide attempters and family member informants. Parents may be more apt to have information about easily observable phenomena (e.g., substance abuse, conduct problems) as opposed to nonobservable phenomena such as emotional distress and hopelessness (Velting et al., 1998). Consistent with this observation, in our own research, we found that parents were more aware of their adolescents' suicide attempts than suicidal thoughts (Klaus et al., 2009). Perhaps not surprisingly, we found that predictors of improved parental awareness included adolescents' perceptions of positive family support and parental history of depression. *When considering discrepant reports from adolescents and parents, we recommend giving substantial weight to positive reports from either person.*

STEPS IN RISK ASSESSMENT AND FORMULATION

Two key factors are important when conducting a suicide risk assessment for a teen. The first is to express a caring attitude and a willingness to help. The second is to gather comprehensive information about suicide risk and protective factors from multiple sources (teen, parent, previous provider) using multiple methods of information (interview, observation, standardized assessment).

Express a Caring Attitude and Willingness to Help

A caring, respectful, helpful approach is a cornerstone of training and practice for mental health professionals. In fact, a meta-analysis of 49 youth treatment studies found that several indicators of therapeutic alliance—counselor interpersonal skills, therapeutic alliance with youth, and youth willingness to participate in treatment—were significant predictors of outcomes (Karver et al., 2006). The effect sizes for these indicators were in the small to moderate range, which suggests a modest yet clinically meaningful impact on outcomes.

When meeting with a teen who may be at elevated risk for suicide, we recommend that you *make it a priority to listen to the teen and try to understand his or her experience, including the experience of pain and hopelessness.* Reflective listening with regular validation of the teen's feelings can help with developing a therapeutic alliance and, ultimately, gathering needed risk assessment information and helping the teen. That is, it is extremely important to listen to and hear the teen's story before asking what may come across as routine and probing risk assessment questions.

Although, to our knowledge, data are not available concerning the impact of therapeutic alliance on the treatment outcomes of suicidal teens specifically, a collaborative and caring approach is uniformly recommended by experts in the field. For example, "maintaining a collaborative, nonadversarial stance" is one of the 24 core competencies agreed upon by the team of experienced suicidologists who developed the *Assessing and Managing Suicide*

Risk core curriculum (Suicide Prevention Resource Center, 2008). One of these suicidologists, David Jobes, previously discussed the importance of the therapeutic relationship when working with suicidal patients (Jobes & Maltsberger, 1995) and has specifically emphasized its continued importance in the approach he refers to as Collaborative Assessment and Management of Suicidality (CAMS; Jobes, 2006). Furthermore, working within a cognitive therapy framework, Ramsay and Newman (2005) carefully delineated the significance of a rich understanding of the client's suicidal behaviors in the context of therapeutic trust following a suicide attempt.

Given the emphasis placed on establishing rapport and a therapeutic alliance in training mental health professionals, why address the issues of "caring attitude" and "therapeutic alliance" in this book? We discuss these here because clinical practice with suicidal teens can be fraught with tensions for the clinician. As discussed in the Introduction, one of the most common tensions is that between the clinician's desire to (1) establish strong rapport and take a collaborative, therapeutic approach, and (2) feel in control and manage the teen's safety. These sometimes go hand in hand, such as when the clinician and teen work collaboratively on a crisis response plan or safety plan (see Chapter 5), or when the clinician and teen agree that a brief hospitalization for stabilization will be beneficial to longer-term therapeutic gain. At other times, however, they may run counter to each other. Realistic fears and anxieties related to the teen's safety and possible suicide risk, in addition to liability concerns, sometimes result in the clinician focusing disproportionately on control. This could result in an overemphasis on safety monitoring and hospitalization as therapeutic strategies. We suggest that it is easier to acknowledge and manage this anxiety to the extent that you can (1) make it a priority to hear the teen's story before focusing on risk formulation and decision making, (2) maintain a collaborative orientation to the teen, and (3) make use of the systematic strategies for risk assessment and formulation described in this book.

Resource limitations can also affect the extent to which a clinician conveys a strong willingness to help. If there are no available inpatient facilities, your agency has few resources to provide after-hours coverage, or there are limited resources for the reimbursement of services, clinicians may be anxious about taking on the care of a suicidal teen. Clinicians in these situations may emphasize the limits to what they can provide rather than convey a willingness to help until the teen's serious problems and concerns are resolved.

What can you do to maintain a caring attitude and clear willingness to help? We recommend the following:

1. When meeting with a potentially suicidal teen, begin by listening to the teen, hearing the teen's story, validating the teen's emotional pain and concerns, and sharing the message that you are interested in helping. This will set the stage for—and contribute to—the comprehensive risk assessment and formulation.

2. Conduct an honest self-assessment of your comfort in working with higher-risk teenage patients and clients. With the systematic strategy and recommendations provided in this book, will you be comfortable working with them through one or more periods of acute risk?

3. Consult regularly with a trusted colleague or supervisor regarding patients and clients at elevated risk for suicide.

4. Assess your attitudes toward individual patients and clients on a regular basis. Maintain the continuity of care whenever possible, but refer the teen to someone else if you detect hostility, rejection, or hopelessness in your attitude and it cannot be quickly resolved following self-awareness.

5. Have ready access to crisis response numbers for emergency services (including police, ambulance, and psychiatry emergency services). Know the procedures for accessing these services as quickly as possible when needed.

6. Be prepared and knowledgeable about your community's outpatient, enhanced care resources for at-risk teens. Familiarity with the options for a higher level of outpatient care (e.g., multidisciplinary collaborators on a treatment team, partial hospitalization programs, case management or wraparound services; the Suicide Prevention Lifeline: 800–273–TALK) may help to diminish anxiety about managing

safety concerns, reduce an overemphasis on overly restrictive levels of care, and, in so doing, convey genuine confidence in our ability to be helpful to a distressed teen and his or her family.

Gather Comprehensive Information about Risk and Protective Factors

Mental health professionals are frequently challenged to gather comprehensive information in a relatively short period of time. Depending on the demands and policies of your agency or practice, it is possible that you will have only 45 minutes or 1 hour, perhaps less, to obtain information on which to base your risk formulation. Because time can be limited, it is extremely important to assess for suicide risk, including suicidal intent and impulses, early in the interview (after listening to and validating the teen's story and experiences), which allows ample time for follow-up if needed. Furthermore, if a teen does seem to be at elevated or perhaps even high acute risk, additional time is taken for the evaluation due to safety concerns, even if it means notifying and rescheduling a waiting client.

CLINICAL NOTE

Because time may be limited for risk formulation, it is extremely important to assess for suicide risk early in the interview.

As described in Chapter 2, risk factors can be conceptualized into three primary categories. We need to gather clinical information about (1) *demographic risk factors*, (2) *clinical risk factors*, and (3) *contextual and interpersonal risk factors*. Moreover, as illustrated in Figure 4.1, a comprehensive suicide risk assessment requires us to delve deeply into the teen's *current and previous suicidal thoughts, impulses, and behaviors*, and to assess the teen's *current mental status*. The tables in Chapter 2, **Risk Factor Checklist for Teen Suicidal Behavior and Suicide (Appendix**

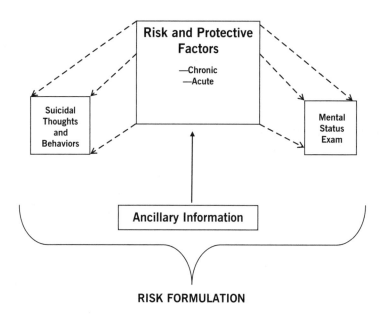

FIGURE 4.1. Risk formulation model, illustrating the areas of inquiry and information gathering for the risk assessment.

A), Questions to Ask about Suicidal Thoughts (Appendix D), and Teen Suicide Risk Assessment Worksheet (Appendix E) are provided for your use as interview and information-gathering guides during a comprehensive risk assessment.

> **Risk and Protective Factors**
>
> - Assess three domains:
>   1. Demographics;
>   2. Clinical (adolescent and family history);
>   3. Contextual, interpersonal.
> - Consider presence, acuity, severity, impairment.
> - Integrate information from ancillary sources and multiple informants.

THE INTERVIEW AS
A PRIMARY RISK ASSESSMENT STRATEGY

Information about risk and protective factors may be gathered using a variety of developmentally sensitive techniques, including interviews, behavioral observation, and psychometrically strong rating scales (American Academy of Child and Adolescent Psychiatry, 2001). Ideally, the risk assessment strategy incorporates multiple informants (e.g., teen, parent/guardian, previous clinical provider) and multiple methods of assessment (e.g., clinical interviews, rating scales, record of previous behaviors). The *clinical interview with the teen*, however, is the cornerstone of the assessment. *It is not possible to conduct a meaningful risk assessment and formulation without conducting a clinical interview with the teen.*

A clinical interview with one or more significant others, such as the teen's parents, is also extremely important. The parent or other informant can provide additional essential background information (developmental history, school history, family psychiatric history), information about the presenting problem and its history, and comprehensive information about the teen's previous treatment history. Furthermore, these individuals are sometimes a key to learning about the teen's suicidal thoughts and behaviors. Even though teens are more likely to report their suicidal thoughts and behaviors than their parents (Brent, Kalas, Edelbrock, & Costello, 1986; Klaus et al., 2009), in some instances teens fail to report their history of suicidal behavior, and the parent or guardian becomes a key informant. Recent research suggests that this occurs with nearly 10% of teens who have positive suicide attempt histories and are hospitalized due to acute suicide risk (Klaus et al., 2009). In other instances, the interviews with significant others can verify and enrich the sometimes limited information provided by the teen. These significant others have observed the teen in different settings or contexts across time, and each can offer a unique perspective and interpretation of events (Achenbach, McConaughy, & Howell, 1987).

Interview Strategies: Gathering Information about the Three Key Domains

Suicidologists are often asked if there is a recommended suicide risk assessment tool for adolescents, one that would enable the mental health professional to gather information about all important risk and protective factors, tally the results, and determine level of risk. Unfortunately, such a tool does not exist. Despite the tragedy that each suicide represents, suicide continues to be a statistically rare event, and therefore, difficult to predict with accuracy (Pokorny, 1983). It is not possible to weigh a series of risk factors and come up with an accurate number that reflects overall risk. Although suicidal behavior is much less rare than suicide, it also poses a problem of prediction. This is partially due to its infrequency and partially due to the unique constellation of risk and protective factors that make up the risk equation for each teen. Across a young person's developmental trajectory, various risk and protective factors intertwine and change over time. In such a transactional model of suicide risk (King, 1997), the risk formulation for each teen is unique.

It is possible, however, to use interview guides that serve to remind us to cover all relevant areas during our risk assessment interview with the teen and parent or guardian. There are several such guides available. One might use the **Risk Factor Checklist for Teen Suicidal Behavior and Suicide (Appendix A)** and the **Teen Suicide Risk Assessment Worksheet (Appendix E)**. In using the Teen Suicide Risk Assessment Worksheet, it is important to note that this is not intended to be a structured interview, but rather a template for information that needs to be obtained and a suggested sequence of questions. The mental health professional asks sufficient questions (or obtains ancillary information) to address the items in each section while conducting the interview with a caring attitude and collaborative approach. *It is an "unstructured" or "semistructured" interview in that the client rather than the interview guide takes center stage.* If it appears that the mental health professional is hurrying to get through a checklist or focusing more on the checklist and the goal of completing paperwork than on the client, it becomes much less likely that sensitive and possibly important information will be forthcoming from the teen.

CLINICAL NOTE

If it appears that the mental health professional is hurrying to get through a checklist or focusing more on going through a risk assessment checklist and the goal of completing paperwork than on the client, it is probably much less likely that sensitive and possibly important information will be forthcoming from the teen.

Specific Inquiry: Suicidal Thoughts and Behaviors

The assessment of suicidal thoughts, impulses, and behaviors should be *conducted relatively early in the interview*. If the teen reveals current suicidal impulses or intent—or chronic and unrelenting suicidal thoughts—substantial time will be needed to fully understand risk and determine appropriate next steps. This will also be necessary, though much less "convenient," if the teen first notes suicidal impulses with a hand on the doorknob at the end of the session. That said, the mental health professional does not need to open the interview with these questions. Depending on the interview context and setting, these questions are sometimes asked within the series of questions involving assessment of mood and depressive symptoms. Alternatively, they are asked as part of the more formal mental status exam (discussed on page 86). If someone is being interviewed in an emergency setting for a psychiatric complaint, these questions may be an initial focus of the interview.

Overall Interview Strategy

There is no single recommended strategy for conducting this interview. Although research on adolescent suicide has proliferated over the past 20 years, it has not focused on specific interview strategies and the sequencing of questions. As such, we rely on "best practices," which we defined in the Chapter 1 as ". . . integration of the best available research with clinical expertise in the context of patient characteristics, culture, and preferences"(APA Presidential Task Force on Evidence-Based Practice, 2006, pg. 273).

One recommended strategy is a three-part assessment of the following: current suicidal ideation/impulses and behavior (precipitating emergency department or outpatient visit or hospitalization), recent history of suicidal ideation and behavior (past few weeks or few months; time frame is client-driven), and lifetime history of suicidal ideation and behavior. The first step in this strategy is asking the teen about his or her suicidal thoughts, impulses, and recent behaviors in a clear and direct manner. Doing so may immediately give the teen the message that we are comfortable talking with him or her about these thoughts and impulses, and that the clinician is not going to avoid or minimize this primary problem and the importance of the teen's safety. Possible questions might include: "How often (and for how long each time) have you been thinking about suicide this past week?" "Have you been thinking about or feeling an urge to harm yourself or end your life this past week?" Additional sample questions are provided in the box on page 83 ("Sample Questions to Ask about Suicide").

A second recommended interview strategy has been put forth by Shawn Shea (1998a, 1998b, 2002). This strategy divides the teen's history of suicidal thoughts and behaviors into four segments: presenting events (past 48 hours), recent events (past 2 months), past events (pertinent suicide-related events that may affect formulation), and immediate events (e.g., suicidal ideation during interview). Although we do not have specific comparative data to argue that one interview strategy is superior to the other, Shea argues that this strategic approach is nonthreatening, clear, and likely to yield the most valid information possible. Regardless of approach, it is important to assess the teen's present status and anticipated status in the near future prior to the close of the interview.

The mental health professional needs to *stay focused on conducting a full suicide-specific inquiry*. Perhaps not surprisingly, some teens will provide a vague or unclear response when asked about suicide. A teen might respond to an initial question such as,

> **Specific Inquiry: Suicidal Thoughts and Behaviors**
>
> - Conduct a suicide-specific inquiry relatively early in interview.
> - Assess current, recent, and previous history of suicidal thoughts, impulses, and behaviors.
> - Assess antecedents, consequences, and "function" of suicidal thoughts, impulses, and behaviors.
> - Assess exposure to suicidal behavior and suicide within family, peer group, and community.

"Have you had any thoughts of suicide or killing yourself during the past few weeks?" with the response, "Not really." It is not possible to know what "not really" means without further inquiry. It is recommended that an initial question such as this be asked at least three times in three somewhat different forms. In addition, it is recommended that any response such as "not really" be followed up with a response such as "Not really?" or "Would you tell me more about that?" or "I wonder if you would be willing to share with me what types of thoughts about death, dying, or suicide you have experienced." or "You answered my question about suicide with 'not really,' which leaves me wondering whether you may be thinking about suicide."

CLINICAL NOTE

If an adolescent responds "not really" to an inquiry regarding suicidal thoughts, the clinician can respond with one of the following:

"Not really?"

"Would you tell me more about that?"

"I wonder if you would be willing to share with me what types of thoughts about death, dying, or suicide you have experienced."

"You answered my question about suicide with 'not really,' which leaves me wondering whether you may be thinking about suicide."

Although this applies to interviews concerning all sensitive or potentially sensitive topics and is not unique to suicide-specific interviews, it is essential for the mental health professional to be comfortable asking these questions. In a sense, the mental health professional indicates—via questions and nonverbal communications—that it is okay and possible to talk about this difficult topic.

CLINICAL NOTE

The mental health professional indicates—via questions and nonverbal communications—that it is okay and possible to talk about the difficult topic of suicide.

If the mental health professional is anxious about asking about suicide or conducting an interview regarding suicide risk, it may be helpful to seek professional consultation and/or role-play the interview with a colleague for desensitization. Greater clinical experience asking these questions may increase the comfort level over time.

Sample Questions

When discussing sensitive topics with teens, it may help to begin with entry questions and "normalize" teen concerns. For example, the interviewer could begin with an initial or entry question about morbid or suicidal ideation and preface it by saying, "Sometimes, when teens are feeling really down, they begin to have thoughts like 'I wish I had never been born,' or 'I wish I was dead.' Have you ever had thoughts like that?" By prefacing the question with information about other teens, the interviewer is indirectly communicating that such thoughts can be a typical or even expected reaction to low mood, thereby reducing the shame that the teen may be experiencing as a result of his/her problems managing current difficulties. While it can be comforting and reassuring to teens to have their feelings normalized, the interviewer must be cautious not to suggest that suicide is an acceptable or common option for

---

Sample Questions to Ask about Suicide

- "I wonder if you've been so down that you've had thoughts about death or wishing you were dead?"
- "It sounds like you've been feeling really down. How often do you feel so down that you feel like hurting yourself?"
- "Do you ever get images or pictures in your head of your own death?"
- "How often do you feel so down or in so much pain that you think about or consider suicide?"
- "Do you sometimes have an impulse to kill yourself? How often do you have such an impulse and when (where, under what circumstances) do you most often have this impulse?"
- "How long have you been thinking about suicide? When did you first begin to have suicidal thoughts?"
- "How long do the thoughts last? How hard is it to get them out of your mind?"
- "Have you had thoughts about how you would do it?"
- "What thoughts or plans do you have?"
- "Have you taken steps toward this plan?" (The clinician may want to follow up with a more specific question; e.g., if a plan was shared to overdose, "Have you ever taken out a pill bottle?")
- "Is there any part of you that wants to die?"
- "Do you have an intent to die?"

---

teens struggling with life difficulties. The clinician must also convey that suicide is a topic he or she is comfortable talking about. If the clinician begins with entry questions about death and dying, he or she needs to move to direct questions about suicidal thoughts and behaviors.

SELF-REPORT QUESTIONNAIRES

Some adolescents may be more likely to share their suicidal thoughts or history of suicidal behavior via a self-report rating scale.

Although such scales are "tools" and not a replacement for the clinical interview, they may serve to prime or enhance the interview between clinician and teen. As discussed in Chapter 2, some adolescents are more likely to report sensitive thoughts and behaviors on rating scales (or on computer surveys) rather than to an adult interviewer (Pealer, Weiler, Pigg, Miller, & Dorman, 2001). The primary tasks for the clinician are as follows: (1) to review the teen's responses before the teen leaves the clinical setting, (2) to follow up on any statements concerning suicidal ideation or behavior that are endorsed by the teen, and (3) to clarify any discrepancy between information the teen reports on the rating scale and in the clinical interview.

CLINICAL NOTE

Self-report questionnaires assessing the adolescent's suicidal ideation and behavior are "tools" that supplement the clinical interview. When using these, the clinician's primary tasks are:

- To review teen's responses before the teen leaves the setting.
- To follow up on statements that the teen endorses.
- To clarify any discrepancies between what the teen reports on the questionnaire and in the clinical interview.

One self-report rating scale that may be useful is the Suicidal Ideation Questionnaire–Junior (SIQ-JR; Reynolds, 1987), which, as described in Chapter 3, has demonstrated excellent psychometric properties in younger and older adolescents. It is easy to read, has 15 items, and can be completed by teens in 2 to 3 minutes. Although the SIQ-JR has shown evidence of predictive validity for suicidal thoughts and attempts across a 6-month period following hospitalization (Huth-Bocks et al., 2007; King, Hovey, Brand, & Ghaziuddin, 1997), more recent analyses with a larger sample of psychiatrically hospitalized boys and girls indicate it may have predictive validity for girls only (King et al., 2012). Especially among boys, a failure to report suicidal ideation on the SIQ-JR does not necessarily indicate the absence of risk for suicidal behavior.

The SIQ-JR could be given to teens with other forms or questionnaires on a clipboard in the waiting room prior to the interview or while interviewing the teen's parents. Alternatively, it could easily be completed by the teen during the actual session. If done in a sensitive way that doesn't interfere with developing an alliance, this approach enables the clinician to provide context for the assessment prior to giving the teen the rating scale to complete. Finally, because the SIQ-JR does not include a question regarding history of suicide attempt, it is recommended that the clinician supplement it with a series of questions assessing whether the teen has previously engaged in suicidal behavior and, if so, the types of suicidal behavior and circumstances under which it occurred.

Similarly, the Beck Scale for Suicide Ideation (BSS; Beck, Steer, & Ranieri, 1988) and the Beck Hopelessness Scale (Beck & Steer, 1988; Beck, Weissman, Lester, & Trexler, 1974) warrant consideration. These scales have good psychometric properties when used with adolescents (Steer et al., 1993a, 1993b). The 21 items of the BSS were based on a semistructured interview and require approximately 5 minutes to complete. The BSS is unique in its capacity to measure both active and passive suicidal ideation. In testing, subjects using this measure reported more severe suicidal ideation than the clinician ratings, suggesting that this may be a more thorough and accurate measure of suicidal ideation.

The Beck Hopelessness Scale (BHS; Beck & Steer, 1988) includes 20 true–false items that assess negative expectations about the future. It requires approximately 2 to 5 minutes for completion and has excellent psychometric properties (Goldston, 2003). Relative to the BSS, the BHS has been used more extensively with adolescents. Higher scores have been associated with treatment dropout in adolescents (Brent et al., 1998). They have also been found to predict suicide attempts among adolescents who have a prior history of suicide attempt (Goldston et al., 2001). The BSS and BHS are relatively easy to use and interpret. Similar to the SIQ-JR, these instruments should be supplemented by a clinician interview regarding previous suicidal behavior.

THE MENTAL STATUS EXAM

Our observations of the teen are a critical part of a comprehensive risk assessment. The mental status exam is based on our interactions with and observations of the teen. As explained below, mental status exams occur upon our first contact with a teen but are also frequently repeated at subsequent contacts, allowing us to observe changes over time. Below, we provide examples of each component of the mental status exam and link this information to the risk assessment process.

Appearance

A teen's appearance may provide information as to his or her level of functioning, identity, and social context. Observations of appearance may include style of dress, hygiene, grooming, jewelry, tattoos, scars (e.g., evidence of cutting or drug abuse), weight, and any odors. A teen's style of dress may provide clues as to peer-group affiliation, identity, and method of self-expression. Teens who present with some unusual aspect of appearance may be at greater risk for bullying or peer rejection. Additional clues to a teen's mood and functioning may be gathered by careful attention to his/her

**Components of
the Mental Status Exam**

- Appearance
- Behavior and attitude
- Motor functioning
- Speech and language
- Mood/affect
- Thinking and perception
- Insight and judgment
- Cognitive functioning

appearance over time. For instance, if a teen who is usually well dressed with careful attention to hygiene comes to an appointment and is noticeably unkempt, this change may be an indication of anhedonia, fatigue, or other symptoms of depression. One must be careful not to draw firm conclusions from appearance changes alone, but should weigh these observed changes in the context of other sources of information.

CLINICAL NOTE

Less attention to appearance may be a result of depression, which is a risk factor for suicidal behavior and suicide.

Behavior and Attitude

Assessment of behavior begins at the moment you first see the teen. In outpatient practice, observations of the teen client or patient in the waiting room can be important. For instance, is the teen curled up and lying down, or talking with animated, pressured speech? Does he or she engage easily with you as the examiner? Is he/she defiant and irritable with parents? Should there be any form of behavioral disturbance, this may influence the clinician's risk formulation. For instance, in an emergency setting, if the clinician notes, "patient was belligerent to his parents throughout the exam, he yelled 'screw you' and interrupted his mother on several occasions," this may be evidence of a mood disturbance (irritability), may signal difficulties in the parent/child relationship, or may be evidence of significant impulsivity. Each of these possibilities are important to consider in developing the risk profile, disposition, and safety plan. In contrast, a teen who engages easily, expresses a desire for help, is cooperative and friendly, and who appears close to and in good communication with parents may be at a lower level of acute risk. Moreover, these observations may guide disposition planning as they suggest a better chance that the parent could appropriately monitor this teen's safety on an outpatient basis.

Motor Functioning

The teen's level of activity, rate of movements, mannerisms and description of any abnormal movements such as a tic, tremor, or posturing should be observed. Psycho-motor retardation or agitation can be indicative of severe depression; similarly motor agitation/hyperactivity may signal ADHD or a manic episode. Evidence of impulsivity, including substance abuse and aggression toward others, is also critical to a suicide risk assessment.

Speech

Rate, rhythm, and tone of speech are commonly assessed in the mental status exam. If a teen is speaking quickly in a hostile, agitated tone, the clinician may be alarmed and consider whether this problem has implications for the teen's level of risk. Should a teen present with incoherent or slurred speech, a drug screen or medical workup may be necessary. Ascertaining from parents whether the behavior represents a change is important. If this is the "normal" way the teen speaks, it may not be as clinically relevant as a teen for whom this was a recent change.

CLINICAL NOTE

Obtain collateral information from the teen's parents when assessing speech and motor activity. For instance, you could ask the parent, "I notice that your daughter is speaking quite quickly. Is this similar to how she usually talks, or is this new?"

Mood/Affect

Mood is the client's or patient's description of his or her emotional state. To elicit information about a teen's current mood, one can simply ask "How do you feel?" or "On average, how would you describe your mood over the last week?" Some teens struggle with putting their feelings into words and are not very descriptive. It can therefore be helpful to provide multiple-choice options (e.g., "Have you been feeling down, so-so, or fairly happy this week?") or to have the teen rate his or her mood on a scale of 1–10. Particularly, if a teen reports feeling severely depressed or anxious, and/or hopeless and in despair, our concern for risk would increase.

Affect generally refers to the clinician's description of the client's or patient's emotional state. In assessing affect we may pay particular attention to the teen's nonverbal communication and the match between presentation and verbal report of mood. Does the teen display a range of emotional responses, or does affect appear blunted? Is the teen tearful? Current level of distress and agitation are helpful when making a judgment about acute risk.

Thinking and Perception

Thought content refers to the information reported by the teen and may include suicidal or homicidal thoughts, delusions, and important topics or conversational points. A teen who shows signs of delusional thinking may have an increased risk due to an altered mental state. Future-oriented thinking may be useful to note as a possible positive sign.

The organization of a client's or patient's thinking is described in the thought process section of the mental status exam. A teen's thought process may be logical and goal directed, or it may be disrupted. Most teens will have a coherent thought process but if a teen cannot consistently form coherent sentences, intoxication, a medical concern, psychosis, or mania may be indicated. This teen may have an impaired sense of reality and would be at increased risk for suicide.

Teens experiencing perceptual disturbances, including auditory or visual hallucinations, often have a psychiatric diagnosis and are at an elevated risk for suicide. Evidence of a perceptual disturbance may include the observation that a teen is responding to internal stimuli (e.g., looking for something that others do not see or turning his/her head as if hearing or seeing something) or a report about the experience of hallucinations. When a patient has difficulty deciphering reality, he or she would inherently be at elevated risk. Of particular concern are command hallucinations encouraging self-harm.

Insight and Judgment

Insight refers, in part, to the degree of understanding the teen has for his or her condition. Some teens have very good insight. They may recognize how their diagnosis or risk profile affects them, and they understand the need for treatment. Other teens have very little insight and either refuse treatment or resist engaging in the assessment process. Insight can also vary developmentally, with younger teens tending to think more concretely and with less self-awareness.

Judgment involves how reasonably a patient reacts in situations. Good judgment entails sound and logical decision making based on what a reasonable person would do in a similar situation. Like insight, judgment can be assessed in the clinical interview through careful listening. Attention to how the teen describes solving everyday and stressful problems will guide the clinician in assessing a teen's judgment. When faced with stressful life events, limited judgment or reduced capacity to see a range of potential options, including positive ways of coping, may elevate risk of suicidal behavior.

CLINICAL NOTE

A teen's judgment or behavior under duress can be very informative. Limited judgment or less capacity to see a range of potential options, including positive ways of coping, can further increase risk in teens during times of increased stress.

Cognitive Exam

Clinician observations about the teen's orientation, level of alertness, memory, concentration, and fund of knowledge can provide information about current intoxication or possible functional impairment due to learning, attention, or true cognitive limitations. Concerns in these areas may point to the presence of academic stressors and/or possible problem-solving deficits.

INTEGRATING INFORMATION TO FORMULATE RISK

When formulating risk, we consider all available information about risk and protective factors (Chapter 2), with particular consideration of the factors that are key to determining level of acute risk: (1) current suicidal thoughts, impulses, and behaviors; and (2) current mental status. It is important to keep in mind that, even following the most thorough risk assessment, it is not always possible to predict which teens will attempt or die by suicide and when they might chose to do so.

There is no formula for determining the level of acute risk or for predicting the likelihood of suicidal behavior or suicide. We offer the examples in the box on page 92 as general guidelines only. It is not an exhaustive list of the many combinations of factors that may place a teen at differing levels of acute risk. Furthermore, although informed by the empirical research on risk factors, the specific categories of high, moderate, and low acute risk have not been empirically validated. Different mental health professionals, including expert suicidologists, may draw the lines between these categories in different places. These examples have been adapted and extended from those included in the Assessing and Managing Suicide Risk (AMSR) training curriculum (Suicide Prevention Resource Center, 2008). In this curriculum, high acute risk is defined as follows: "A person who has recently engaged in a potentially lethal suicide attempt or taken actions in preparation to kill himself or herself is at high acute risk for suicide. A person who is experiencing persistent ideation with a strong intent to die by suicide or a suicide plan is at high acute risk for suicide" (p. 50).

Appendix G, SAFE-T Card, is a resource to help the clinician recall the components of a comprehensive risk assessment,

Levels of Acute Risk

HIGH ACUTE RISK

- Suicidal intent (any level of positive intent) *plus* a suicidal plan that includes specific method.
- Suicidal intent (any level of positive intent) *plus* preparatory actions (such as securing firearm or securing materials for suffocation).
- Suicidal ideation *plus* history of multiple suicide attempts *plus* high levels of hopelessness and impulsivity *plus* alcohol intoxication.
- Chronic, unrelenting suicidal thoughts *plus* command hallucinations (to hurt self) *plus* availability of means.

As is evident from these examples, there are many combinations of factors that result in the designation of high acute risk. **The key is the potential for self-harm in the immediate future.**

MODERATE ACUTE RISK

- Chronic suicidal ideation *plus* history of multiple suicide attempts.
- Bipolar disorder with periods of impulsivity and potential self-harm.
- History of single suicide attempt *plus* current major depressive episode.
- Substance use disorder *plus* difficulty coping with stress and negative affect *plus* a high level of hopelessness.

LOW ACUTE RISK

(Note: This is not an insignificant level of acute risk. However, in these instances, there is no evidence of suicidal intent or a suicidal plan.)

- Chronic, low level of suicidal ideation (occasional thoughts of suicide with no plan and no intent) plus depressive disorder.
- Single Axis I disorder such as bipolar disorder, major depressive disorder, substance use disorder, panic disorder, posttraumatic stress disorder.
- History of suicide attempt 1 year ago but no current Axis I disorder and no currently elevated level of hopelessness, agitation, or impulsivity.

formulation, and disposition plan: (1) identify risk factors; (2) identify protective factors; (3) inquire about suicidal thoughts, behaviors, plans, and intent; (4) determine risk and intervention approach; and (5) document. The Suicide Assessment Five-step Evaluation and Triage (SAFE-T) card was originally conceptualized by Douglas Jacobs, MD, and developed in collaboration with Screening for Mental Health, Inc., and the Suicide Prevention Resource Center.

Special Considerations: Assessing and Formulating Risk in an Acute Care Setting

Clinicians who work in acute care settings experience a number of unique challenges that warrant special consideration. In these settings, teens are frequently at highly elevated risk and in acute distress. Such distress can negatively affect the teen and/or parents' ability to provide clear and comprehensive information. In addition, the teen's reluctance or fear of being hospitalized may influence his or her responses to a clinical interview. Taken together, these factors suggest that a calm, patient, and systematic approach to risk assessment and formulation is indicated. This can be especially challenging because the clinician is likely seeing the teen for the first time. It is not possible to understand the current crisis in context and to compare the teen's current level of functioning with the teen's baseline functioning. To further compound this challenge, the emergency care may be taking place after hours, limiting access to sources of information that would otherwise be available.

The emergency setting can be one of the busiest places for a mental health clinician to practice. High-stakes decisions (to hospitalize or send home) must often be made within a relatively short time frame. Despite the time pressure, safety remains a primary concern. Given the multiple challenges of conducting a risk assessment and formulation in these settings, listening carefully to the teen and family and taking a systematic approach to risk assessment and formulation is particularly critical.

> **Challenges of Risk Assessment in an Emergency Setting**
>
> - The patient/family may be in crisis.
> - There is no previous rapport between clinician and patient.
> - The clinician lacks context or information about baseline level of functioning or recent history.
> - There is limited time to make an assessment.

Factors to Be Considered in Hospitalizing Teens with Acute Suicide Risk

First, it is important to note that a teen's level of acute risk may change from the time the teen presents to the emergency setting to the time when the risk formulation is completed. This is especially true when, during the risk assessment interview, stressors are removed, rapport is established, and the evaluation and conversation are therapeutic. For instance, empathic listening and validation of the teen's experience, exploring reasons for living, and collaboratively developing a safety or crisis response plan (as described in Chapter 5) may be sufficient to reduce an acute level of risk. If, however, a teen continues to be at acute suicide risk, a decision must be made regarding the safest and least restrictive treatment setting. Depending on the resources available in the area, teens may be referred to an inpatient psychiatric hospital, partial hospital or day program, or outpatient mental health treatment. The decision to hospitalize is made with a full consideration of the applicable state laws for mental health treatment. State mental health codes are highly variable. In some states, minors can only be admitted with a parent or guardian's consent. Other states allow a physician to hospitalize a patient under emergency conditions. Most states define criteria for admission in terms of harm to oneself or others; however, each state interprets this meaning differently. It is therefore essential for the mental health clinician to be familiar with state laws and practices. If this information is unclear, it is best to contact an attorney or administrator at the school, hospital, or agency who may be able to offer guidance.

A careful and accurate risk assessment and formulation guides a clinician in making a decision regarding the possible appropriateness of hospitalization. Unfortunately there are no steadfast rules or "litmus tests" as to when we should hospitalize a teen (see Chapter 5 for an additional discussion of a practice parameter and guideline concerning hospitalization). As described above, a teen may be at acute, high risk but may not be verbalizing suicidal ideation or a suicide plan. For instance, Johnny is brought to the emergency department by his parents. Although Johnny denies suicidal thoughts, his parents share that Johnny's friends reported he sent a text message that he doesn't know why he is alive and is actively thinking about ways he could kill himself. Johnny is not getting out of bed and has started drinking again. This situation is similar to the last time he attempted suicide. In this scenario, hospitalization may be warranted even though Johnny is not actively sharing suicidal thoughts. There are other instances when a suicide plan is reported and inpatient admission is not the only option for maintaining the patient's safety.

Risk factors that include active delirium, florid psychosis, or acute intoxication suggest the need for psychiatric hospitalization (Martin & Volkmar, 2007). Similarly, teens who remain aggressive or agitated, or who have failed treatments in less restrictive environments, may need psychiatric admission. Discharge may be a more reasonable option if the teen's parents understand the risk and safety concerns and are willing, able, and available to actively participate in safety planning. Should the parent display behaviors or make statements in the emergency setting leading you to question his/her capability of taking on the responsibility, then this information should be factored into your decision. Parents' inability to secure the environment or restrict lethal means tend to support the need for hospitalization in the short term as a safer alternative to returning to an environment in which the teen has ready access to lethal means.

> **Factors to Be Considered in Hospitalizing a Teen at Elevated Risk**
>
> - Level and acuity of risk.
> - The safest and least restrictive treatment setting.
> - State mental health codes related to being at risk of harm to self or others.

CLINICAL NOTE

A discharge home from the emergency department may be a less reasonable option if the parents do not feel safe taking the teen home—you should take into account the parent's condition, understanding, and his or her capability of taking on responsibility when considering discharge.

In summary, when conducting a risk assessment in an acute care setting, the clinician must make a decision regarding hospitalization or discharge home while facing a number of challenges to obtaining accurate and valid information. Given these challenges, it is particularly important to use the systematic approach described earlier in this chapter.

DOCUMENTING AND COMMUNICATING RISK FORMULATION AND PLAN

Regardless of the type of setting—acute care or outpatient—careful documentation and communication of findings are essential. From a clinical point of view, documentation serves the following purposes: (1) a quality assurance self-assessment for the clinician who conducted the risk formulation, (2) a communication to other professionals who are caring for the client (or will be in the future), and (3) a record of contacts. **Appendix F, Documentation of Teen Suicide Risk Assessment**, is a documentation form or template for clinicians.

When we document our assessment and risk formulation, we review what we have learned and integrate this information. If we have neglected to gather pertinent information, we generally become aware of it at this time. This two-step process, conducting and then recording the risk assessment and formulation, provides us with feedback about the quality and comprehensiveness of our work. Of equal importance, the written record enables other health professionals and clinicians who are caring for the teen to benefit from the information that is provided and to coordinate efforts. This is extremely important for effective practice. Adolescents at elevated risk for suicide may share their suicidal thoughts or impulses with one provider and not another. Shared information enables us to close this potential gap, essentially wrapping a protective and informed network of professionals around the at-risk teen. Similarly, timely information sharing enables professionals who are caring for the teen to work together with consistent recommendations and follow-through. Finally, careful and timely documentation serves as an excellent clinical record that we can refer to when needed.

From a legal point of view, there is no evidence that a clinician completed the risk assessment and formulation unless it is recorded in writing. Careful documentation may decrease the possibility of malpractice liability in the unlikely event that a suicide occurs. It may also be essential for full reimbursement for services.

CLINICAL NOTE

From a legal point of view, there is no evidence that a clinician has completed the risk assessment and formulation unless it is recorded.

When to Document

Documentation should occur immediately following the interview or assessment session with the adolescent who is at elevated risk for suicide (within 24 hours and preferably sooner). This is the case even if we do not believe we were able to gather all of the information we would have liked for a comprehensive risk assessment and formulation. For instance, perhaps the adolescent ran from the office and refused to respond to additional questions. Or perhaps you are awaiting a key document to be sent to you from a previous provider or the inpatient unit where the adolescent was recently hospitalized. Perhaps you neglected to conduct key components of the mental status exam and are suffering from the hindsight that sometimes occurs after a patient or client leaves the office and the clinician has a nagging feeling that something was missed. We must record the best information we have at the time. The key is to integrate the available information, to formulate risk, and to devise a plan of action. When additional information becomes available, it is added as a new entry into the record (all entries must be dated and timed) and, if appropriate, a new formulation and plan of action is developed and recorded at that time.

What to Document

The content of your documentation should clearly indicate that you conducted a risk assessment and thoughtfully integrated the information to formulate risk and develop a plan of action. (Additional information on the "plan of action" is addressed in Chapter 5.) This means that the documentation will have at least two major components: (1) information about risk and protective factors, and (2) your formulation—judgment about level of acute risk with your rationale for this judgment, which is based on an integration of risk assessment information. It is not sufficient to name risk and protective factors and then provide your plan of action (e.g., safety plan and continued outpatient therapy). This documentation of suicide risk assessment and formulation is best thought of as one component of your full evaluation or session documentation.

The documentation may be formatted in a number of ways. Your clinic or facility may have a required form with sections for recording types of information (risk factors, protective factors, formulation, plan); you may be encouraged to write a "free-form" paragraph, as shown on the next page, or you may want to create

---

Sample Documentation

Sarah has several risk factors for suicidal behavior. She currently meets criteria for bipolar disorder II, she reports that she occasionally uses alcohol and "drinks too much," she has a definite history of sexual abuse, and she has a history of one suicide attempt (ingestion of approximately 12 aspirin) approximately 1 year ago. Moreover, the specific assessment of her current suicidal thoughts and impulses indicated that she thinks vaguely about killing herself about once or twice a week. Nevertheless, Sarah indicates that she has no suicidal intent and has not had any suicidal intent or thought about any suicidal plan during the past several months. She reported that she "feels safe" and that when she "drinks too much," it is "with friends" and has not been associated with negative moods or thoughts of self-harm. The mental status exam also revealed that she is thinking clearly and coherently, is not delusional, and is able to consider options and problem solve at this time. It also indicated that she is not feeling emotionally overwhelmed at this time. In addition to these positive indicators and her reported sense of good connectedness to others, Sarah's openness to discussing her personal struggles and her interest in treatment seem to be strengths. In summary, despite the risk factors noted above, given these strengths and the fact that she is not currently and has not experienced any suicidal intent for several months, she is judged to be at low to moderate risk at this time. Therefore, the plan is to work with her on an outpatient basis at this time with twice-weekly appointments and frequent monitoring of her suicide risk status.

---

your own subheadings and make use of bullet points rather than sentences and paragraphs. It is the content that is critical.

Communicating/Sharing Risk Formulation and Plan with Others

After determining that a teen is at risk, it is important to communicate the nature of the risk and to alert key persons in that teen's life or other providers involved in the teen's care. If, following a comprehensive risk assessment, it is determined that a child needs to be referred to a higher level of care (e.g., emergency department or admission to an inpatient psychiatric facility), clinicians are strongly encouraged to coordinate this referral with either a telephone call, a written release of records (with parent permission), or both. This is especially important when the referring clinician has known the youth for a length of time and can provide needed information about baseline levels of functioning and historical context to the emergency department and/or inpatient treatment teams.

When an at-risk teen is being managed on an outpatient basis, good communication and collaboration allows family members and other professionals to have a heightened level of awareness and to participate more fully in the safety plan (described in Chapter 5). They can also alert the clinician to any observed changes in the teen's risk status. It is important to get a release of information form signed by the parent or guardian before sharing the information. It may be important to share it with the primary care doctor, a school social worker, or the teen's therapist or psychiatrist at another agency.

Sharing the risk formulation with the teen's *primary care physician* can be as simple as forwarding a copy of the recent note, but often a telephone call and conversation is helpful. Such communication may take time, but, if possible, will add value to the clinical care. The primary care doctor may be familiar with the family and able to partner with the clinician in the process of ongoing risk assessment. The primary care doctor can be encouraged to continue the risk assessment process by asking about suicidal thoughts at each encounter and to share any additional information with you that might be pertinent to the teen's risk status.

In clinical practice with teens, the *therapist and psychiatrist* are not always located at the same agency or office setting. It is often necessary to take steps to communicate bidirectionally with other providers. With the teen's and parent's or guardian's permission, this may be done via a phone call, especially in those situations in which the risk is the highest, or by sharing written records of evaluations and treatment plans. Teens may selectively share information about their suicidal thoughts. By sharing the findings that lead to the determined level of risk, care providers can assure that they are informed and in alignment with the treatment planning and care.

Communication with the *school* can also be helpful. The school social worker or counselor will often have longitudinal information about the teen's behavior, academic functioning, peer relationships, and overall mental status that can be helpful for the risk assessment. In addition, if there have been concerns observed in the school setting, school officials may feel uneasy about the teen's safety. By communicating the risk assessment and giving the school a role and specific goals in this process, they often feel more at ease after gaining a sense of direction. More information is provided in Chapter 6 regarding strategies for working effectively with schools.

One of the most important people to communicate with is the *parent/guardian*. Open communication regarding risk with the teen's parents/guardian is essential. This topic is covered in detail in Chapter 6. Parents usually have the most frequent contact with the teen and are therefore key to ongoing risk assessment and monitoring. Communication and collaboration with parents is critical regardless of the care setting: discharge from an inpatient unit, discharge to home or outpatient care following an emergency department visit, or management by an outpatient therapist or psychiatrist. These communications can provide an opportunity to educate parents about suicide risk and care management by sharing information about warning signs, creating a safe home environment, and increasing support for their child. Unfortunately, too many parents have the experience of departing from a mental health or psychiatric evaluation of their child, being told to "watch him," but feeling unsure of what they are watching for or how to help should they grow concerned again.

During ongoing treatment, the parent must continuously be kept informed about the clinician's current understanding of the teen's risk and contributing factors. For instance, if depression and drug use are factors, the parents should be aware of these so they can partner with the clinician to monitor these aspects of the teen's well-being. Parents generally appreciate some education on what they can do in this process.

CONCLUSION

In this chapter, we have reviewed basic principles of risk assessment and formulation, emphasizing the overall approach, guidelines for conducting a suicide-specific clinical interview, and the supplementary role of self-report questionnaires. Factors influencing the decision to hospitalize were reviewed along with challenges to assessment in an acute care setting. Examples of documentation and appropriate communication were provided.

CHAPTER FIVE

Intervention Planning and Care Management

CHAPTER OBJECTIVES

▶ Delineate the three components of an intervention plan:

- Immediate interventions for safety;

- Short-term interventions for support, enhanced monitoring, and facilitation of effective coping;

- Treatment for ongoing suicide risk, psychiatric disorders, and psychosocial concerns.

▶ Describe the importance of repeated risk assessments.

▶ Describe the importance of follow-up on referrals and missed appointments.

▶ Discuss the value of continuing education, consultation, and collegial support.

In this chapter, we describe and illustrate the primary components of an intervention plan for suicidal adolescents, emphasizing the importance of immediate and short-term interventions
focused specifically on suicidal thoughts and behaviors, in addition

to ongoing treatment for suicide risk, Axis I psychiatric disorders, and other presenting problems such as bullying and severe parent–teen conflict. We also describe the importance of repeated risk assessment, follow-up on all referrals to other providers, and follow-up regarding missed appointments. Finally, because clinical work with suicidal teens and their families can be highly stressful and because we have only limited empirical evidence to guide us in the care management of suicidal teens, the importance of continuing education is emphasized. This is particularly crucial because a number of clinical studies are currently under way, and we anticipate that new information will become available about best practices in intervention and care management. In the meantime, we recommend that clinicians carefully consider the existing evidence; continually monitor key outcomes with each suicidal adolescent under their care; make clinical judgments based on an understanding of each teen's presentation, history, and environmental circumstances; and seek consultation.

INTERVENTION PLANS FOR TEENS AT ELEVATED RISK FOR SUICIDE

Although we do not have definitive scientific evidence to guide intervention planning with potentially suicidal teens, our prioritization of safety concerns and our knowledge about the effectiveness of treatments provide important clues to what should be included in a tailored intervention plan. These include *immediate interventions* and *short-term interventions*, in addition to treatments for the teen's diagnosed condition(s) and ongoing psychosocial problems.

Immediate Intervention Plan

The immediate intervention plan delineates what we intend to do immediately and within the first 24 to 48 hours after the suicide risk has been identified. An important consideration is whether the clinician, based on the risk assessment and formulation, determines that *hospitalization* is required. If the clinician identifies "acute high risk," as discussed in Chapter 4, hospitalization should be considered and is likely appropriate. The *Practice Parameter for the Assessment and Treatment of Children and Adolescents with Suicidal Behavior*, published by the American Academy of Child and Adolescent Psychiatry (AACAP) (Shaffer & Pfeffer, 2001), recommends psychiatric hospitalization for children and adolescents after a suicide attempt if their "unstable condition makes behavior unpredictable, indicating at least short-term serious risk" (p. 38S). Possible indicators include psychotic symptoms, current intoxication, a history of multiple serious suicide attempts, and an inability to develop a therapeutic alliance with the clinician. These guidelines also support hospitalization for children and adolescents who have engaged in suicidal behavior and for whom there is a lack of sufficient collateral history, adequate supervision upon discharge, or a secure environment (e.g., removal of firearms, securing medications). As stated in the guidelines, "Being aware of one's limitations in prediction and influence over the family will promote a cautious approach" (Shaffer & Pfeffer, 2001, p. 38S).

The National Institute for Health and Clinical Excellence (NICE) in England and Wales has also published guidelines for the clinical care of children and teens who engage in self-harm and are under the age of 16 years, noting the special needs and vulnerabilities of this age group (NICE, 2004). In these guidelines, self-harm is defined irrespective of purpose or intent, and includes suicide attempts as well as nonhabitual behaviors that cause harm (e.g., ingestions, self-injury, self-mutilation). Taking a more cautious approach than the AACAP Practice Parameter, these guidelines recommend overnight admission to a pediatric ward for all youth who have engaged in self-harm so that the clinical care team can complete a comprehensive risk assessment and develop a clinical care plan. These guidelines note that alternative placements, such as psychiatric hospitalization, may be required depending on a variety of factors that include, but are not limited to, child protection issues, physical and mental health of the child or teen, and time of presentation. These guidelines also emphasize the importance of involving clinicians who have specialty training to work with children, adolescents, and families; who are skilled in risk assessment;

and who have regular supervision and access to experienced consultation. Finally, similar to the AACAP Practice Parameter, the NICE guidelines emphasize the importance of a full assessment that extends beyond the child or adolescent's presenting problem to include the family, the child or adolescent's social functioning, and child protection issues.

The key commonalities of these two sets of guidelines are the emphasis on a comprehensive risk assessment and formulation that takes into account developmental and family issues. To the extent that it is possible to accomplish this in an outpatient clinic or emergency department, an overnight stay may not be necessary. That is, the immediate intervention plan may not entail hospitalization if there are no indicators of suicidal plans or preparatory action steps, and if the clinician judges the level of acute risk to be in the low to moderate range. This may be the case even if the teen is characterized by several significant underlying or chronic suicide risk factors.

When hospitalization is not pursued for a teen who presents with suicide risk, other immediate interventions are still recommended as safeguards. These steps include (1) *provision of a tailored crisis contact card* (see example on page 107); (2) collaboration with the teen to develop a crisis response or *safety plan*; and (3) a *conjoint session with the teen and parent(s) or guardian(s)* to discuss "red flags" for possible increased suicide risk; an immediate plan for increased structure, support, and safety monitoring; and the importance of removing access to lethal means. In some

---

Immediate Interventions for Safety

- Consider hospitalization (ascertain level of acute risk; clinical judgment based on comprehensive risk assessment and formulation).
- Develop safety plan (crisis response plan).
- Provide crisis contact card to teen and parent(s)/guardian(s).
- Conduct session with parent(s) and teen.

instances, as discussed below, there may also be a separate meeting with the teen and/or parent to address some of these issues.

Crisis Contact Card

We recommend that all clinicians who work with suicidal teens consider developing and using their own crisis contact cards. These cards can be given to teens and parents or guardians with an explanation of the card's contents, taking the time to address any questions or concerns. Some clinicians print or write this information on the back of their business card; others prefer to print separate cards for this purpose. The information to be included on the crisis contact card could include the following:

- 911 (emergency)
- Local emergency services center location and number
- 1–800–273–TALK (8255) (Suicide Prevention Lifeline)
- Clinician's name and phone number (hours available at number)
- Parent's/guardian's name and phone numbers

It may be helpful to have the teen call a number (e.g., national crisis line) with the clinician in the office as a supporter and facilitator. This may serve to desensitize the teen to making a similar type of call in the future.

Safety Plan

Safety plans, versions of which have been referred to as crisis response plans (Jobes, 2006; Rudd, Joiner, & Rajab, 2001), are recommended as immediate interventions for individuals of all ages who are at elevated risk for suicidal behavior and suicide (Rudd et al., 2001; Stanley & Brown, 2008; Suicide Prevention Resource Center, 2008). The primary objective of these plans, which are developed collaboratively with the client or patient, is to help the client identify what he or she can do when experiencing suicidal thoughts or impulses (Rudd, Mandrusiak, & Joiner, 2006). These plans may be integrated as needed into the ongoing treatment of individuals at elevated risk for suicide (Jobes, 2006; Rudd et al., 2001; Stanley et al., 2009; Suicide Prevention Resource Center, 2008) or function as stand-alone interventions, as has been described by Stanley and Brown in their work in emergency settings (Stanley & Brown, 2012).

Although we have almost no data to validate the essential components of safety plans or crisis response plans, to validate the extent to which teens use them, or to validate their usefulness in reducing suicidal behavior, these plans have a solid theoretical and empirical rationale. They can assist teens in identifying their personal cues or triggers for increased suicide risk, and they incorporate a range of coping strategies to help suicidal teens manage their emotional distress and suicidal thoughts and impulses. These strategies are central components of empirically validated psychotherapies for suicidal adults, particularly cognitive-behavioral therapy (CBT; Brown et al., 2005) and dialectical behavior therapy (DBT; Linehan et al., 2006). These strategies are also one component of both the emergency department intervention for suicidal adolescents that was developed by Rotheram-Borus, Piacentini, Cantwell, Belin, and Song (2000) and are associated with an improved outcome when used in combination with a CBT family treatment and the Collaborative Assessment and Management of Suicidality (CAMS; Jobes, 2006). Furthermore, they have been recommended by an interdisciplinary team of expert suicidologists, the Clinical Skills Core Competency Curriculum Committee, which developed the Assessing and Managing Suicide Risk (AMSR) training curriculum (Suicide Prevention Resource Center, 2008) that is being distributed nationwide via the Suicide Prevention Resource Center (*sprc. org*).

We recommend including multiple components in a safety plan for teens. These components are adapted from and generally consistent with components that have been recommended by suicidologists who have been involved with developing and implementing a nationally disseminated training curriculum (Suicide Prevention

Resource Center, 2008) or conducting large-scale clinical trials (Stanley et al., 2009; Stanley & Brown, 2008). The components are as follows: (1) a list of or statement regarding the teen's personal triggers for heightened risk of self-harm or suicide; (2) a list of coping strategies that the teen generates with the clinician through a process of brainstorming and guided discovery; (3) a list of individuals who are sources of healthy support, with names and contact information; (4) clinician contact information; (5) crisis contact numbers, including for emergency services; (6) a statement about limiting access to suicide attempt methods (lethal means); and (7) a place to record one or more "reasons for living." The teen and the clinician sign the safety plan, which may also be signed by the parent or guardian.

It is recommended that the safety plan include a distraction coping strategy (which for teens may include music, computer time, television, phone call to friend, shopping) that may help the teen tolerate distress and get away from problems in the short term. Safety plans may also include a physical activity coping strategy that is both distracting and highly engaging (e.g., jogging, aerobic exercise, biking, spinning), and an individually tailored cognitive coping strategy that involves self-statements (e.g., "I'll feel better when I get past final exams next week," or "I have people who care for me and can help me through this"). In the safety planning intervention described by Stanley and Brown (2012), the client or patient is asked to consider internal coping strategies as a first step in effortful coping (following recognition of warning signs).

The process of developing the safety plan also encourages the teen to make use of a support system of family, friends, and professionals. The safety plan includes a place to record the names of two to four individuals whom the teen feels are supportive and whom the teen would be comfortable calling and talking with for support when upset. By including the contact information for support persons within the safety plan, one possible barrier to using the support system is eliminated. Finally, these plans will include crisis contact information such as the information that is included on the crisis cards, described earlier, and a statement regarding the importance of removing access to suicide attempt methods.

A sample safety plan is provided in Figure 5.1. The clinician individually tailors the safety plan through a collaborative brainstorming process with the teenager. As part of this process, the clinician assesses the teen's readiness to use the safety plan and discusses with the teen anticipated barriers to its use. Many teens already have one or more strategies they use to cope with high levels of distress, self-harm impulses, or "suicide triggers." If there has been a recent suicidal incident, the clinician can brainstorm with the teen about why the teen didn't use one of these strategies or contact a support person prior to the incident. Through a collaborative process, the clinician works to facilitate the teen's consideration of how to decrease barriers and increase the likelihood of using the safety plan in the future. A blank **Safety Plan Form** is provided in **Appendix H** for your use.

Conjoint Session with Parent and Teen

One of the first steps in partnering with the parent for the teen's safety is to *openly communicate to the parent that there is elevated risk for suicidal behavior.* Sometimes the parent is completely unaware that the teen is experiencing suicidal thoughts or that he or she has previously engaged in suicidal behavior (Klaus et al., 2009). If a teen shares this information with a clinical provider, it becomes the provider's responsibility to be sure that the parent is aware of the suicide risk. It is important for the clinician to share his or her judgment concerning the level of this risk. Clear and direct communication should be used. The clinical provider can share the factors that led her to the conclusion that risk is elevated in addition to factors that are not currently present but might also increase risk, should they develop.

We recommend meeting with the parent and teen together to communicate this concern, encouraging the teenager to share the information directly unless there are strong contraindications such as intense parent–teen conflict that would make it difficult for the

Safety Plan Form

1. What are my triggers for suicidal thoughts or self-harmful behaviors? How might I recognize when I need to take steps to protect my well-being and remain safe?

   Triggers—when I feel really stressed. Recognize—when I find myself hiding out
   in my room and not talking to anyone.

2. The steps I will take when I experience these triggers, suicidal thoughts, or self-harm urges:

   a. Try to relax by *listening to music, using my headphones*

   b. Do something physically active such as *going for a run*

   c. Distract myself by *watching sports or a movie on tv*

   d. Use coping statements (thoughts) such as *"I have some good friends who care*
   about me" and "This is just a bad day, tomorrow will probably be better."

   e. Contact a family member, friend, support person:

Name	Phone Number
Grandma	*xxx–xxx–xxxx*
Jeremy	*xxx–xxx–xxxx*
Mark	*xxx–xxx–xxxx*

   f. Call my therapist or emergency numbers OR go to emergency department:

   Emergency: 911

   Local emergency services: *xxx–xxx–xxxx*

   My clinical provider/therapist: *xxx–xxx–xxxx*

   (Times I can reach my clinical provider) *Mon–Fri 8:00 a.m.–5:00 p.m.*

   Suicide Prevention Lifeline: 1-800-273-TALK (8255)

   g. Move away from any method or means for hurting myself; involve family member or support person in limiting my access to means.

(continued)

FIGURE 5.1. Safety plan for Jason, a 13-year-old male who resides with foster parents due to a history of physical abuse by his biological parents. He presents with aggressive behavior, poor emotional regulation, and major depressive disorder.

3. A couple of things that are very important to me and worth living for are:

hanging out with my friends

being there for my little brother

Signed:

Jason	_9/20/12_
Client	Date
Emilie	_9/20/12_
Therapist	Date
Jackie	_9/20/12_
Parent/Guardian (if possible)	Date

FIGURE 5.1. (*continued*)

parent to hear the information in the teen's presence. If the teenager is uncomfortable doing so or there are strong contraindications to doing so, the clinical provider can communicate the information to the parent and invite the teen to be present so there is an opportunity to clarify what was said and share additional information. This is sometimes easier for the teen to do after the topic has been raised. However, even if information is shared with the parent(s) individually, some work with the teen and parents together is usually beneficial for discussing and successfully implementing an agreed-upon safety plan to prevent suicidal behavior.

We recommend *talking with parents about the importance of restricting access to potentially dangerous suicide attempt methods* because accessibility to these methods, which are commonly referred to as lethal means, is an established suicide risk factor. This discussion may take place during discussion of the teen's safety plan, as this is one component in safety planning. Providing parents with psychoeducation in the emergency department about the importance of restricting access to lethal means has been associated with parental actions to restrict such access in their homes (Kruesi et al., 1999; McManus et al., 1997). It may be best to do this with the parents alone so that teens do not inadvertently learn about or begin to consider potential suicide attempt methods. However, if teens are collaborating with the parent and clinician in working toward their own safety, it may be beneficial to talk with the teen about removing possible suicide attempt methods such as medications and razor blades. This may enhance safety by making it less likely that methods will be accessible during an acute suicidal crisis. If additional time or complicated steps are needed to access a suicide attempt method, the teen who is in an acute suicidal crisis may calm down and/or change his or her mind. A clinician colleague has described an instance wherein a boy was on a chair with a noose around his neck and ready to kick the chair away. His cell phone rang and he decided to pick it up. After talking to his friend, he changed his mind and took the noose down. This example highlights the transient nature of some suicidal crises and the potential preventive impact of lethal means restriction.

The parent should be provided with information about warning signs for possible increased risk. One suggested approach is to provide the parents with a handout on suicide warning signs and to discuss these warning signs together (see **Appendix I, Suicide Warning Signs for Parents**). In addition to monitoring for these signs, the parents can be empowered to help monitor both mood and suicidal thoughts. Some parents are uncomfortable discussing the topic of suicide with their teen. In this case, the clinician can help the parent by providing specific suggestions for how to ask questions about mood and suicide. Parents might feel more comfortable asking the teen how his or her mood is on a scale of 1–10 or asking about suicidal thoughts using this same scale. Parents can then monitor for changes over time. Many teens are also more receptive to this form of questioning from their parents, as it starts with a closed-ended question before leading into dialogue. When asked, "How are you feeling today?" a teen may simply groan at the parent or answer with a automated response of "Fine," rather than report a true reflection of his/her mood. That same teen when asked, "On a scale of 1 to 10, with 10 being the most depressed and 0 being not depressed at all, how would you rate your mood?" may respond with a more accurate, albeit short, response.

Short-Term Intervention Plan

A short-term intervention plan focused specifically on suicide risk is recommended as a supplement to the ongoing treatments that target the teen's ongoing psychiatric disorders and psychosocial problems. A short-term intervention plan is recommended because the psychotherapies and psychoactive medications that target the psychiatric disorders and related problems common among suicidal adolescents are not immediately effective. As examples, CBT for depression has not been evaluated as a one-session treatment (Brown et al., 2008; David-Ferdon & Kaslow, 2008); practice parameters for psychoactive medications for depression advise at least 4–6 weeks of adequate dosage before considering alternative treatment strategies (AACAP, 1998); and alcohol and substance abuse often required sustained, multimodal treatment approaches (American Psychiatric Association, 2006). In the interim period, we must take active steps to help the teenager manage his emotional distress and to help the family manage the stressful situation of elevated risk.

One common strategy is to *schedule and conduct more frequent sessions* during this interim period. Although we do not have empirical evidence to guide us, these sessions seem to provide important support to the teen and parent. They also offer opportunities for ongoing risk assessment, a review of any possible side effects associated with medications, active problem solving

---

Short-Term Intervention Options

- More frequent sessions:
  - o Provide support;
  - o Engage in problem solving;
  - o Enhance coping skills; and
  - o Monitor risk.
- Provide telephone access to clinician.
- Increase parental monitoring of teen safety.
- Reduce teen's stressors.

---

regarding current problems associated with exacerbated stress and distress, and enhancing coping skills that can serve as an alternative to suicidal behavior. Indeed, increased treatment frequency provides a larger "dose" of therapy in addition to a means for ongoing risk monitoring. The sessions during this intervention phase may focus most heavily on support and active problem solving. The provider can partner with the teenager to consider a variety of possible coping strategies and options. Many suicidal teens have a sense of feeling "stuck," and are relieved to (1) hear from someone that their situation is temporary, (2) know that there are alternative solutions, and (3) have someone help them with problem solving.

A second common strategy during this intervention phase is to *offer the parent and teen more direct access to you, the clinician,* if they feel they need to talk with someone to avert an emergency, such as self-harmful or suicidal behavior. This is consistent with the therapist or counselor being named on the safety plan as one possible contact person when "highly distressed," "upset," or "feeling suicidal." Although it is unrealistic for many clinicians to be available 24 hours a day 7 days a week (clinician quality of life is important too!), the parent and teen should always be able to call someone. Ideally, the clinician will be available during regular office hours and either the clinician or an emergency on-call person will be available at other times. For the highest-risk cases, the clinician may choose to give out direct numbers (e.g., cell phone number) so that he or she can be contacted if necessary and within carefully discussed parameters. Consistent with the strategy used in DBT, clinicians may offer "coaching calls." This involves encouraging teens and parents to call for coaching in the event of a suicidal impulse. The coaching is intended to help teens to use their coping skills as an alternative to suicidal behavior (Linehan, 2011; Miller, Rathus, & Linehan, 2007).

Parents may be enlisted during this phase to partner with the clinician in monitoring the teenager's safety. Strategies include additional support and conversations (if the relationship facilitates this), increased oversight or monitoring, and facilitating the teen's attendance at more frequent psychotherapy sessions. These strategies need to be recommended to the parents; it should not be assumed that all parents will have the personal strength, skills, and follow-through to implement these strategies, or that they will automatically implement these strategies without encouragement.

The parent may also be able to assist by *temporarily lowering or buffering existing stressors on the teen*. For instance, if there is a lot of pressure related to homework and grades, lowering the expressed demands can help. A parent might contact the school or teachers in this process or simply lessen the emphasis on home-work. Another example may be to temporarily relieve the teen from a chore or responsibility. The clinician can facilitate an open conversation between the parent and teen about what might be helpful. Many times, the teen will offer the most helpful suggestions. However, when parents inquire, they should be prepared to follow reasonable suggestions.

Increased monitoring is an important component to safety, but a delicate balance of monitoring and appropriate levels of autonomy is needed in order to maintain an alliance with the teen. At home, the parent may increase monitoring by checking in with the teen more often. If the teen is in his/her bedroom, this form of checking in should be done with an observation rather than by talking through a closed door, as the teen may be doing something of concern that he/she will not reveal through a short conversation alone. Ideally, this is conducted as part of a collaborative agreement with the teen during this intervention phase, which minimizes the experience of intrusion and loss of autonomy.

Limiting a teen from going out with friends can be appropriate if the teen's friends have a negative influence and the parents don't trust them. However, teens also depend on support from or even just fun times with friends to overcome a stressful period. Some teens may become more distressed if cut off from communication or spending time with friends. In this way, it is helpful for parents to use their best judgment by taking into account their teen's past behaviors with friends, and the knowledge and trust the parent may have of the particular friend. Increased monitoring may mean that the teen has to check in more often, that they are not allowed to be with certain friends, or may not be able to spend as much time out. Parents should be made aware of both the complexity and importance of decisions related to monitoring their teen. Decisions should be made on a case-by-case basis. The clinician can show support and help the parent through this process.

Treatments for Psychiatric Disorders and Psychosocial Problems

The clinician's comprehensive evaluation commonly indicates that the suicidal teen has one or more psychiatric disorders in addition to significant psychosocial problems such as peer victimization, a troubled parent–teen relationship, or a history of sexual abuse. The clinician must prioritize these treatment targets and consider the existing evidence base for appropriate treatments. The specific treatments; the possible sequencing of treatments; and issues of dosing, frequency, and intensity are generally recommended by the treatment provider and then discussed with the parent and teen in a collaborative manner. Because the evidence base for most treatments is still developing, safety considerations and other issues of cost–benefit are real (e.g., required number of sessions per week, financial cost), and family values are an important consideration, the clinical provider often discusses more than one treatment option with the family.

A review of possible treatments for suicidal adolescents is beyond the scope of this book due to the heterogeneity of these teen's presenting problems (e.g., bipolar disorder, major depressive disorder, conduct disorder, alcohol dependence) and the importance of tailoring treatments for each teen based on a comprehensive risk assessment and formulation. Nevertheless, there has been a concerted effort in our field to develop effective interventions that are specifically designed for suicidal adolescents, and research with adults suggests the value of specifically targeting the suicide risk in psychotherapy (Brown et al., 2005). Unfortunately, however, in a meta-analytic review of 17 quasi-experimental and experimental (randomized controlled designs) studies of targeted interventions for adolescents who presented with suicidal thoughts or behaviors, findings indicated that these interventions are only slightly effective in helping suicidal teens feel less suicidal (in terms of suicidal thoughts) and may actually increase self-harmful and suicidal behavior over the long term (Corcoran, Dattalo, Crowley, Brown, & Grindle, 2011). It should be noted that this analysis of longer-term outcomes was based on a small number of studies with outcomes spanning 6–18 months. Overall, the review indicated that interventions specifically developed for suicidal adolescents have demonstrated little benefit over usual clinical care. These disappointing findings may be partially due to the heterogeneity of the suicidal adolescents who were included in these studies and their variable treatment needs.

One of the most promising recent studies focused on the treatment of suicide risk among a somewhat more homogeneous subgroup of suicidal adolescents with co-occurring substance abuse (Esposito-Smythers, Spirito, Kahler, Hunt, & Monti, 2011). In a randomized clinical trial enrolling 40 adolescents recruited from an inpatient psychiatric hospital, Esposito-Smythers and colleagues found that an integrated outpatient cognitive-behavioral intervention was more effective than enhanced treatment as usual in reducing heavy drinking days, days of marijuana use, global impairment, number of emergency department visits, and suicide attempts. Additional clinical trials are needed that target the treatment needs of specific subgroups of suicidal adolescents.

THE IMPORTANCE
OF REPEATED RISK ASSESSMENTS

Assessments should be conducted on an ongoing basis. A teenager's level of risk for suicidal behavior and suicide is not static. A basic risk assessment, with inquiries regarding suicidal thoughts (range of thoughts? intent? plan?), should be conducted and documented at each session. Furthermore, there are certain situations and indicators that call for a comprehensive assessment and reformulation of risk. These include (1) a change in treatment setting or plan, such as discharge from a psychiatric hospital, which is associated with elevated suicide risk (Meehan et al., 2006); (2) a change in treatment provider; (3) emergence or exacerbation of a major stressor in a teen's life; and (4) an abrupt change in a teen's behavior or mental status, including but not limited to expression of suicidal thoughts.

CLINICAL NOTE

The following situations call for a comprehensive assessment and reformulation of risk:

1. A change in treatment setting or plan, such as discharge from a psychiatric hospital.
2. A change in treatment provider.
3. Emergence or exacerbation of a major stressor in a teen's life.
4. An abrupt change in teen's behavior or mental status, including but not limited to expression of suicidal thoughts.

THE IMPORTANCE OF FOLLOW-UP FOR NO-SHOWS AND REFERRALS

One last safety consideration involves the clinician's response when the patient and his or her family do not show for a scheduled appointment. Follow-up is essential whether this appointment was a follow-up appointment with the primary treating clinician or a referral to a consulting psychiatrist or other provider. Should an appointment be missed, the clinician should contact the parent/guardian by phone to discuss. While sometimes it may be due to a change in the teen's schedule, an illness, or unintentional error, follow-up can still be helpful. It serves the following functions: (1) the clinician demonstrates a caring attitude and commitment to the plan of care, (2) the clinician has an opportunity to check in and learn whether something has occurred that suggests possible elevated risk and need for an urgent evaluation, and (3) it provides an opportunity to schedule the next visit to ensure continuity.

CONTINUING EDUCATION, CONSULTATION, AND COLLEGIAL SUPPORT

New evidence continues to emerge to guide our interventions with suicidal teens. For this reason, it is critical to establish a process for continuing education and ongoing professional development. The Suicide Prevention Resource Center (SPRC) provides a wealth of updated information as well as a Listserv to notify members of recent developments in the area of suicide prevention (*sprc.org*). The annual conference sponsored by the American Association of Suicidology (AAS) provides another opportunity to update knowledge of best practices in assessment, intervention, management, and prevention of suicide risk. In a joint effort, the SPRC and AAS worked together to develop a clinical competencies curriculum that is being nationally disseminated in a 1-day workshop format, "Assessing and Managing Suicide Risk." Additional information about this curriculum is available at (*www.sprc.org/trainingin-stitute/amsr/clincomp.asp*) and a related 2-day curriculum, "Recognizing and Responding to Suicide Risk," sponsored by AAS, is also available (*www.suicidology.org/training-accreditation*). As studies continue, we will gain more information about necessary components of immediate and short-term interventions as well as the interface between suicide-specific interventions and those designed to target the teen's diagnosed condition.

Clinical work with suicidal teens and their families can be highly stressful. It can be helpful to establish avenues for collegial support and consultation on difficult cases. Providers who work in hospital and clinic settings that make use of a team approach often have built in avenues for both personal professional consultation and case consultation (for a second opinion). Providers in private practice settings can establish their own consultation group, following established ethical guidelines concerning information sharing and confidentiality.

CONCLUSION

In this chapter, we have reviewed the need to develop immediate and short-term intervention plans that are specifically tailored to a particular suicidal teen. Immediate interventions (conducted within the first 24–48 hours after risk status is determined) may include a psychiatric hospitalization, use of a crisis contact card, development of a safety plan, and collaboration and communication with parents. Short-term interventions may include more frequent therapy sessions, ongoing assessment and safety monitoring, and a focus on coping, problem solving, and emotion regulation. Continued collaboration with parents related to safety monitoring is also critical. We conclude the chapter by encouraging clinicians working with suicidal teens to obtain peer support, consultation, and continuing education owing to the difficult nature of working with suicidal teens as well as to the need for emerging data to guide current practice strategies.

CHAPTER SIX

Partnering with Parents and Schools

▶ Discuss strategies for working effectively with parents, including developing a partnership, providing education and resource materials, and striking an effective balance between teen confidentiality and safety.

▶ Discuss how to deal with several of the most common questions and challenges that arise when working with suicidal teens and their parents.

▶ Discuss what schools can be encouraged to do to help suicidal teens.

▶ Describe strategies for working effectively with school personnel.

In this chapter, we describe how clinical providers can work effectively with parents and school personnel to help the teen who may be suicidal. We describe the benefits of creating strong communication and a working alliance with parents whenever possible; provide further recommendations for educating parents about suicide risk; discuss the balancing act between adolescent confidentiality and adolescent safety; provide examples of treatment plans developed in partnership between providers, teens, and parents; and describe and provide suggested solutions to several common challenges that emerge in clinical work with suicidal teens and their parents. We also discuss how clinical providers can work effectively with schools and parents to care for a suicidal teen's needs while they are in the school setting. We describe components of a recommended partnership between clinical providers and parents, clinical providers and schools, and among clinical providers, parents, and schools. A collaborative approach is emphasized and resource materials are provided for the reader.

STRATEGIES FOR WORKING EFFECTIVELY WITH PARENTS

Alliance and Partnership

As is the case with many forms of mental health treatment, adolescent outcomes are improved when parents are involved and supportive of the treatment plan (e.g., Barrett, Dadds, & Rapee, 1996; MTA Cooperative Group, 1999). It is especially critical that mental health providers establish a strong alliance and working relationship with the parents of teens at risk for suicide because, as discussed in Chapter 5, we must often enlist parents to increase their level of supervision and monitoring of an at-risk teen in order to ensure his or her safety.

It is understood that there may be factors that make this challenging or limit the extent to which we can establish a strong working relationship (e.g., parental substance dependence, abusive relationship between parent and teen, parent who is overwhelmed with minimal emotional resources). In these instances, we involve the teen's parent(s) or guardian(s) to the extent that is feasible and beneficial. When parents are not able to be a therapeutic presence in their teen's treatment, it can help to involve another adult such as a grandparent or other family member to support the teen's treatment and recovery. Our recommendations offered below for involving parents could easily be applied to another supportive adult in the teen's life.

At a most basic level, an alliance with parents is critical because it is usually parents who fund treatment (via their insurance or out-of-pocket payments), who must provide permission for treatment of a minor in most states, and who usually schedule the treatment appointments and provide transportation to them. Furthermore, parents generally are able to provide information about their teen that is important to the comprehensive risk formulation and treatment plan. Parental involvement can also improve treatment adherence and the generalization and maintenance of treatment gains. Many evidence-based psychotherapies involve the acquisition of new skills and behaviors that teens must practice during the week. When parents know what these new skills are and when teens should be using them, they can provide support, encouragement, and reminders to the teens to implement their new skills, thereby supporting therapeutic gains. In addition, suicidal teens may be prescribed some form of psychiatric medication as part of their treatment plan. It is critical that parents be on board with this decision and work actively to promote adherence to the medication regimen as prescribed. These examples of the many ways in which involved parents can actively support treatment underscore the critical reasons for building a strong working alliance with parents.

The most important component to building this alliance is fostering open communication between the provider and parents. Parents should be given an opportunity to share their insights about their adolescent during the initial risk assessment as well as during ongoing treatment appointments. Parents should also be given time to ask any questions that they may have about their teen's risk status or treatment plan. Reciprocally, the provider should provide the parents with information about the regular risk assessment of the teen. Finally, parents should be actively involved in treatment planning.

Educating Parents

Often the first step in developing a plan to manage teen suicide risk is to provide education to parents. Psychoeducational approaches often contain three important components: education, support, and skill building (Klaus & Fristad, 2005). Information about the teenager's psychiatric disorder(s) and related stressors, the impact they have on functioning at home and school, and the pros and cons of different treatment options should all be discussed with parents (as well as the teen). Information about the teenager's specific risk factors for suicide should also be discussed. Support and empathy should be offered by the provider.

CLINICAL NOTE

The following steps foster a strong working alliance with parents of suicidal teens:

1. Actively seek and respect parents' input about their child's functioning and risk status. It is important to hear their perspective.

2. Develop a treatment plan in partnership with parents, providing the rationale for all components and enlisting them to support adherence to the plan.

3. Make sure parents are educated about risk factors, warning signs, and have a clear emergency plan.

4. Offer information to parents about the overall focus and goals of treatment sessions.

5. Provide parents with regular updates about the teen's risk status, alerting them to any concerns regarding possibly elevated risk.

Skill building can include guidance in effective communication and family problem-solving strategies as well as information about how to sensitively talk with their child about his or her suicidal ideation and mood. A number of studies have found benefits of family psychoeducational interventions on outcomes for adolescents and adults with depression, bipolar disorder, and schizophrenia (e.g., Fristad, Verducci, Walters, & Young, 2009; Goldstein, 1978; Miklowitz, et al., 2000; Sanford, et al., 2006). Sometimes parents have struggled to communicate with their teenage child and have questions about how to facilitate improved communication. **Appendix J, Tips for Communicating with Teens**, offers tips for talking with teens about their lives, including their concerns and sensitive topics.

Parents may appreciate specific education and coaching on how to ask their teen about suicidal thoughts. Many parents are very uncomfortable with raising this topic. Some fear that talking about suicide may in some way trigger suicidal thoughts. The clinician can educate the parent that there is no information to support this notion of "suggesting" suicide. In fact, a carefully conducted empirical study identified no negative impacts of assessing for suicidal thoughts (Gould, et al., 2005). This information will be a relief to many parents. You can also help the parent to open lines of communication about this sensitive and anxiety-provoking topic. One way to do this is to have the parent practice asking the questions in session. This will give the clinician an opportunity to actively coach the parent through this process.

In a study of a psychoeducational support intervention for teens who had recently been released from an inpatient hospitalization for suicide risk (King, Klaus, et al., 2009), parents and other supportive individuals in the child's life were provided with a psychoeducational workshop followed by 3 months of weekly consultation. The educational workshop included information about the prevalence of adolescent mental health problems, specific information about their child's diagnosis and treatment plan, education about warning signs for suicide and how to talk to adolescents about safety concerns, and basic tips for communicating with teens. Local crisis resources were also provided. Results suggested that this intervention had very modest positive outcomes for certain adolescents and no negative effects.

Parents whose children have been evaluated for suicide risk often report high levels of anxiety and distress. This anxiety is often compounded when teens are being managed on an outpatient basis, as parents assume a higher level of responsibility for the teen's safety, but may or may not be aware of risk factors, warning signs, or even how to talk with their child about suicide. Although much more research is needed, it is possible that one important benefit of parental psychoeducation may be to address parental anxiety and distress and help parents to be educated consumers in seeking care for their children (Mendenhall, Fristad, & Early, 2009). A plan for parent education must at a minimum encompass the following information: (1) warning signs for suicidal behavior and suicide, (2) language for asking about suicidal thoughts and impulses, (3) crisis contact information and an emergency plan, and (4) discussion of the importance of means restriction. Several family resource guides have been developed across the country as part of the youth suicide prevention efforts funded by the Garrett Lee Smith Memorial Act. Many of these resources and others can be accessed via the SPRC online library (under populations and settings: youth), which is referenced in **Appendix K, Useful Websites.**

The treating clinician should review risk and protective factors as they apply to the individual teen (see Chapter 2) and should work with parents to increase their comfort level in talking with their child about suicide (see Chapter 3, screening for sample questions). Moreover, the safety plan should be reviewed carefully with parents to document that parents have been given a crisis contact card or crisis information and are aware of emergency numbers and local crisis resources, such as the nearest emergency room. Finally, parents should be educated about the importance of means restriction as a suicide prevention strategy.

CLINICAL NOTE

A plan for parent education must at a minimum encompass the following:

1. Warning signs for suicidal behavior and suicide.
2. Language for asking about suicidal thoughts and impulses.
3. Crisis contact information and an emergency plan.
4. Discussion of the importance of means restriction.

Means Restriction

As described in Chapter 2, firearms are the most frequent method used by older teenage boys who die by suicide in the United States, and firearms are used by a significant minority of teenage girls who die by suicide. Because some suicide attempts are impulsive, reducing access to lethal means can serve two purposes: it may postpone the suicide attempt, and in that time the impulse for self-harm may pass and/or the means chosen may be less lethal.

Effective means-restriction education involves working with parents to determine what in the home environment could be used for self-harm and removing the teenager's access to it. In addition to restricting access to firearms, it is recommended that parents restrict access to prescription and over-the-counter medications. Parents can be instructed to begin by surveying their home to locate these medications and then determine which ones are currently in use and unexpired. Any expired medications can be returned to pharmacies for safe disposal (contact your local pharmacy's website for information). The remaining medications can be stored in a locked and "out-of-the-way" location in the home.

The Balance: Teen Confidentiality and Teen Safety

When working with adolescents, mental health professionals always have to balance the importance of protecting privacy (and the alliance with the teen) with the parents' need for information. When working with suicidal adolescents, these issues become even more critical, as parents' anxiety about their children's safety often cause them to request even more information. Most adolescents are striving toward autonomy, and a natural part of this process is the desire to pull back from parents, maintaining more privacy about their thoughts and feelings. In addition, family conflict and the adolescents' perception (accurate or not) that "no one understands me," is a common part of suicide risk, making adolescents even less comfortable including their parents in treatment (Daniel & Goldston, 2009). When clinical providers can effectively negotiate this balancing act, the interests of all parties are better served.

We recommend that clinical providers discuss these issues openly and honestly with teens and parents at the beginning of a treatment relationship in order to establish trust between the teen and provider and between the provider and parent.

Suggested Dialogue with Suicidal Teens and Parents

Provider: We need to discuss how to balance your daughter's desire for some privacy with your very real concerns about her safety and your need for information about how she is doing. In order for your daughter to feel comfortable in treatment, she has to trust that I will protect her privacy and not tell you every little thing she says. On the other hand, as parents, it is important that you trust me as well and know that I will give you updates about how she is doing, what we are working on in treatment, and whether my level of concern for her safety is elevated.

I pledge to you both that I will work with you to strike a balance between these two issues during the course of our work together.

To Teen: I promise you that I will not tell your parents every detail you tell me. I will respect your need for privacy. *But,* I am obligated to talk with your parents if I have any reason to believe that you are in danger of hurting yourself or someone else, or if someone is hurting you. I will also share with your parents any concerns that I have about a change in your risk status—level of risk.

To Parent(s): I will always come to you if I have any concerns about your child's safety. As partners in her treatment, we will all work together to develop the best treatment plan for her and for your family. On a regular basis, I will share with you the progress she is making toward her treatment goals.

Developing a Treatment Plan in Partnership

Following the comprehensive risk assessment and careful work to build an alliance with the parents and the teen, the next step is to set treatment goals and to develop a plan for how to reach those goals. As discussed in Chapter 5, in providing educational information to parents and teens, the provider reviews the teen's diagnosis, the available treatments, and the evidence base supporting them. The treatment plan should include specific goals to alleviate symptoms, reduce risk factors, and increase protective factors for the teen. This will necessarily vary by individual, but may include working to increase positive connections to supportive others, developing improved coping and problem-solving skills, decreasing hopelessness, and reducing substance use or depressive symptoms. It is important for the treatment goals and the plan to reach these goals to be acceptable to both the teen and the parents. Often it is useful to have parents and teens contribute to the goal-setting process jointly or individually.

COMMON CHALLENGING SITUATIONS

Below are some commonly encountered challenges in working with suicidal teens and their parents.

Challenge 1: "My son doesn't tell me anything."

As discussed above, it is common for adolescents to desire privacy and independence from their parents. In these cases, it can help to work with the teen to develop a support system of trusted others who may not be parents, such as a pastor, coach, aunt or uncle, or a family friend. Having a therapeutic relationship with a mental health provider can also be helpful for parents if the teen is more forthcoming with the provider than he or she is at home with parents. Sometimes, a teen's reluctance to communicate with parents may signal difficulties in the home environment or parent–child relationship, and this may be an important focus of treatment and recovery. Parents can be encouraged to (1) accept and support the teen's development of a broader support system of adults; (2) work on strengthening their relationship with the teen, which may involve improving their listening and communication skills; and (3) maintain an open channel of communication.

Challenge 2: "She is just manipulating me. She only wants attention."

Often parents see suicidal statements as attention-seeking or manipulative behavior, and for this reason take it less seriously than perhaps they should. It is true that suicidal behavior can be a means of communicating intense distress and unhappiness. Self-injurious behavior may be the only way a teen can think of to create change in his or her situation. It may be the only way he or she knows how to ask for help. In these cases, developing better methods of communicating about feelings and needs can be a helpful part of a treatment plan. Educating parents about the teen's mental health needs can also open the doors to more effective family communication. If a teen has the capacity to manipulate people or situations, he or she probably has some good cognitive ability and the hopefulness and motivation that goes with trying to "make something happen." These qualities may be strengths for the teen and useful to the therapeutic process.

Challenge 3: "My son refuses to take his medication and won't go to treatment."

This situation can be extremely frightening for parents who are concerned for their child's safety. Often poor adherence by teens to treatment can be a signal of other concerns. Some teens prefer to "speak their mind" through their actions or inactions, as opposed to directly communicating their feelings. Poor adherence can be a sign that the teen does not like or trust his treatment provider or that he or she has not been included sufficiently in the treatment planning or decision making. Parents are encouraged to talk with the teen and, if this is the case, to interview other providers who may "click" better with the teen, as this connection is critical to successful treatment.

It is also common for teens to become frustrated with the slow speed of recovery. For instance, if one of the presenting problems is depression, it may take several weeks for medications and psychotherapy to reduce depressive symptoms. This type of delay of gratification can be difficult for adolescents to tolerate. Moreover, this situation may be exacerbated and even result in increased hopelessness when the treatment that is initially recommended does not seem to be effective and a change in treatment plan must be initiated. It is important to help teens have appropriate expectations for their recovery and for the effectiveness of recommended treatments.

In this context, we conceptualize recovery as significantly improved functioning (less emotional distress, improved functioning with family, friends, and at school) and improved quality of life. We emphasize to parents that we will begin with the treatment or treatments that have the strongest evidence base to suggest they will be effective. However, we note to them that individual tailoring is usually needed over time, as each teen responds differently to these treatments. We also emphasize to parents that we plan to monitor (assess) positive changes and celebrate the teen's progress in treatment and recovery. That is, a "cure" is not the endpoint that we hold out to teens and their parents; as the treatment provider, it can be useful to try to meet the teen where she is, assess her concerns, and help her to move forward in a healthy direction.

Challenge 4: "How do I know this drug is safe for my child?"

Concerns about the safety and efficacy of psychiatric drugs are common among parents. These concerns were heightened following the FDA black-box warning that was placed on the use of antidepressant medications with minors in 2004 and extended to also include young adults in 2007. It is important for providers to be familiar with the research regarding the safety and efficacy of medications that are commonly used to treat children and adolescents. It is also important for providers to be familiar with the evidence base for the effectiveness of medications and/or psychotherapy for the teen's primary problems and diagnosed conditions. This will enable providers to partner with parents, and often the teen as well, in considering their treatment options. Without this information, it is impossible to consider the cost–benefit ratio that characterizes the balance between a treatment's safety and effectiveness profiles. Although our evidence base is continually expanding, one book that addresses these issues for the majority of child and adolescent disorders is *Childhood Mental Health Disorders: Evidence Base and Contextual Factors for Psychosocial, Psychopharmacological, and Combined Interventions* (Brown et al., 2008).

In addition, it can be helpful to be conversant with biopsychosocial models, which liken mental health to physical health concerns. Often, comparing chronic disorders like diabetes or asthma to depression or ADHD can help parents understand the role of medications in treatments (e.g., you would never tell your diabetic child to just "snap out of it," you would give her insulin; having depression is similar, and medications can play an important part in treatment). Helping parents to learn about the biological bases of many mental health conditions can assist in their decision making. Similarly, understanding that the decision to treat pharmacologically is one that may have risks, but that the decision not to treat may also have risks. These critical decisions should be made within a strong partnership between the providers, parents, and teen.

Challenge 5: "What do I do with the parent who regularly searches the Internet for treatment information, seems to double-check all of the information I provide, and tells me about the treatment options?"

This is extremely common, particularly in communities where parents are well educated and Internet savvy and where computer access is readily available. As a positive frame, this behavior suggests interested parents who take initiative and truly want to partner with the provider in figuring out the "best treatment" for their teen. It is sometimes the case that the teens themselves also search online for information about their condition or to find information pertinent to understanding possible treatments and their effectiveness.

It is recommended that clinical providers (1) reward and support the parent and/or teen's initiative in seeking this information, and (2) steer them to the most reliable websites for this information. **Appendix K, Useful Websites,** could readily be copied and used as a handout with teens and their parents. A family-friendly website that is particularly useful for obtaining information about psychotherapy is *www.effectivechildtherapy.com*.

STRATEGIES FOR WORKING EFFECTIVELY WITH SCHOOLS

Because most teens spend 30–40 hours per week at school, it is vital that school staff feel comfortable and prepared to manage teens at elevated risk for suicide. According to the national Youth Risk Behavior Survey (YRBS), approximately 1 out of every 6 or 7 high school students report serious suicidal ideation, 1 in 8 have made a plan to attempt suicide, and 1 in 14 actually made a suicide attempt (CDC, 2012b). School personnel may become aware of a student's suicide risk in numerous ways: through school-based screening and risk assessment, when a student seeks out a trusted teacher or counselor to report distress, when peers report concerns about a fellow student to school staff, when teachers notice a marked decline in the student's functioning, or when parents or someone on the mental health treatment team discloses information about a student's risk status to the school.

In a recent survey of school psychologists conducted by the American Association of Suicidology, 86% of respondents reported that they had counseled a student who had threatened or attempted suicide, 35% reported that a student in their school had died by suicide, and 62% knew a student who had made a suicide attempt and survived (Berman, 2009). Despite the prevalence of suicide risk in our nations' schools, most school mental health professionals and teachers report perceiving themselves to be ill-prepared to respond effectively to a suicidal teenager (Berman, 2009; Miller & Jome, 2008). In the next section, we discuss how clinical providers can work effectively with schools and parents and how the mental health treatment team can effectively work together to care for a suicidal teen's needs in the school setting.

School-Based Services and Resources

More research is needed to guide schools about how best to manage at-risk students, but most authors recommend a "whole-school approach" that includes universal, selected, and indicated

---

What Schools Can Do

- Develop a comprehensive suicide preparation plan that includes universal, selected, and indicated prevention, crisis management, and postvention planning.
- Identify at least one staff person who is highly trained to manage high-risk teens.
- Establish a collaborative care team with the parents and treatment team (or primary clinical provider).
- Work with the collaborative care team to reintegrate and support the teen following a suicidal crisis.

---

prevention, clear crisis management guidelines, a strong referral network with community mental health providers, and postvention services designed to prevent contagion (Berman, 2009; Kalafat, 2003; Kim & Leventhal, 2008; Zenere & Lazarus, 2009). Universal prevention strategies often include education and skills training for adults (teachers, administrators, counselors, etc.) and students regarding recognizing and responding to suicide risk. Zenere and Lazarus (2009) also write about the goal of creating a school culture of safety and respect that encourages students to share their concerns with adults. Each of these preventive efforts will help school staff to feel more prepared and confident in their ability to reintegrate and support a high-risk student. Taking steps to manage a high-risk teen who is returning to school is considered indicated prevention, as these strategies are meant to prevent a completed suicide (Jacob, 2009; Kalafat, 2003).

As discussed above, there are many ways that schools become aware of a student's high-risk status and students may return to their school routine with varying levels of acuity. Some students may be returning from an inpatient hospitalization following a suicide attempt; others may be returning following an emergency department visit for significant suicidal ideation; while still others are returning to school following an outpatient assessment for depression, a related condition, or suicide risk. Regardless of the individual situation, students are best served when caring adults in all settings are on the same page and working together to support that teen's recovery.

There are a number of resources available to school staff to improve the training and comfort level of school professionals in managing adolescents at risk for suicide. Many of these are listed in **Appendix C, Suicide Prevention Resources for Schools (Guidelines and Education/Awareness Programs)**. The Suicide Prevention Resource Center (SPRC; *www.sprc.org*) has a wealth of information designed for school staff as well as a registry of effective programs and practices that can be useful in designing universal prevention strategies (see **Appendix L, Evidence-Based Youth Suicide Interventions**). In addition, the American Association of Suicidology has released an accreditation program to train school staff to be certified school suicide prevention specialists (*www.suicidology.org*).

Programs designed to address risk factors for suicide, such as bullying and harassment related to sexual orientation, are also critical parts of the school's preparation plan to manage high-risk adolescents. **Appendix C, Suicide Prevention Resources for Schools (Guidelines and Education/Awareness Programs)**, includes information about the "Stop Bullying" campaign (*www.stopbullyingnow.hrsa.gov/index.asp*).

The Collaborative Care Approach

Following an inpatient hospitalization or other suicidal emergency, many teens express serious reservations about returning to school. They wonder how to explain their absence or symptoms to teachers and peers and are concerned about the stress of their academic responsibilities. Parents often express concerns about "labeling" their child at school, privacy, and stigmatization by students and school staff. In contrast, school professionals often express grave concerns about how to be most helpful to a student when schools often are not informed of the full extent of the student's difficulties. Teachers and school mental health professionals may feel that they are out of the loop when it comes to a teen's mental health. This can be extraordinarily challenging when that student is spending 30–40 hours per week in the care of school staff.

Although stigma and gossip are real concerns, it is our strong recommendation that mental health professionals and parents form a partnership with school staff to share information and develop a school-based plan that will meet the student's needs during the school day. Schools that have an active suicide prevention/crisis management plan in place may make parents more comfortable and willing to share private or confidential information.

The treating clinician is encouraged to secure a release of information from the teen's parents to allow information exchange with the school. The treating clinician should let someone at school (e.g., classroom teacher, school social worker/psychologist, principal) know about the risk and protective factors characterizing the teen's situation, the acuity of the suicide risk, and the safety planning that has occurred. Similarly, school personnel should be encouraged to share their observations about changes in a student's risk factors, current academic or social stressors, or overall functioning with the clinician and parents. When school staff members are informed about a teen's safety plan, they are able to support the teen's adherence to the plan during the school day. For example, the clinician could (with teen and parent permission) share some of the supportive adults the teen has identified, and school staff could encourage the teen to seek the support of these individuals while at school. Similarly, the soothing or distracting activities that a teen may identify could be shared with school and incorporated into a

---

What Mental Health Providers Can Do

- Obtain two-way release of information from parents to allow communication with the school.
- With parent and teen permission, share information about a student's risk and protective factors, risk assessment, and safety plan.
- Work together to ensure that the school environment is supporting recovery and not adding additional social or academic stresses.
- Help a teen decide what to share and not share with peers at school.

school schedule (e.g., allowed to bring an iPod to school to listen to music in the nurse's office, allowed to spend extra time in the art room drawing). With active and open communication, the treatment team and school can work together to ensure that the teen's time in school is contributing to their recovery process.

It can also be extremely helpful for parents and the treatment team to work closely with the school to modify academic pressures during the recovery period and to provide additional academic supports during the school day. Sometimes these interventions can be done informally, but at other times they must be done formally by qualifying a child for services as a seriously emotionally impaired student. In **Appendix M, Sample Letter to Formally Request School Services**, you will find a sample letter for parents to provide to schools requesting an evaluation and a meeting to discuss possible accommodations. Table 6.1 also provides a list of possible accommodations for suicidal adolescents returning to their school environment.

When a collaborative care approach is under way, the student's reintegration to a school routine can proceed much more smoothly. Ideally, parents, clinicians, and school staff are working together to help the teen to anticipate and plan for the reintegration. If the teen has been psychiatrically hospitalized for suicide risk, the school counselor or other school mental health professional may be able to attend the discharge planning conference at the hospital. If this

---

TABLE 6.1. Possible Accommodations at School for Suicidal Adolescents

- Reduced class schedule/shortened school day.
- Shortened assignments.
- Extensions on major projects or tests that may be contributing to stress.
- Study or note-taking buddy when concentration is impaired.
- Social work services during the school day.
- A flash pass to leave class to see the social worker without having to explain or ask permission—to be used when significantly distressed.
- Use of self-soothing techniques identified in the student's safety plan.
- Access to supportive adults identified in the safety plan.
- Assistance to take needed medications during school hours.

is not possible, a release of information form signed by the parent will enable the hospital staff to discuss with the appropriate school personnel by telephone.

Following a school absence for inpatient hospitalization, teens are often most concerned with what they will tell their peers about where they have been. This decision is a very personal one, but should be guided by the caring adults in that student's life. It is ironic that at the time when teens most need support and connections to others (and often believe most strongly that no one cares about their situation), it is difficult for others to support them due to the culture of secrecy and stigma that surrounds suicide and suicide risk (Pompili, Mancinelli, & Tatarelli, 2003). Often peers, teachers, and other adults in a teen's life want to help but are not sure what to say or do. Creating a community of caring people around that high-risk teen during reintegration to school can be an important part of treatment.

CONCLUSION

This chapter emphasizes the importance of collaborative relationships between clinical providers, the parents of teenagers, and school personnel. The clinician's partnership with a teen's parents can facilitate the comprehensive risk assessment and evaluation, the sharing of education and resource materials, safety monitoring, family support of the teen, and adherence to the treatment plan. Extending the network of supportive and caring adults further, this chapter described how clinicians can also work effectively with school personnel and how parents and school personnel can communicate with each other and help suicidal teens.

CHAPTER SEVEN

Legal Issues

CHAPTER OBJECTIVES

▶ Discuss the legal considerations involved in working with suicidal youth.

▶ Provide guidelines for how to minimize your risk of legal problems.

Fear of legal ramifications is common when working with individuals who are at elevated risk for suicidal behavior and suicide. This fear is not entirely unfounded, as clinicians who work with suicidal teens are at a higher risk of being sued than those who do not work with high-risk groups. In fact, attempted suicide and suicide are among the more common reasons for litigation involving psychiatric patients (Simon & Shuman, 2009). Although no clinician is immune from the possibility of being sued (Packman & Harris, 1998), the good news is that the fear of a potential lawsuit is much more prevalent than the actual risk of ending up in a courtroom. This chapter is designed to provide you with relevant information about legal risk as well as suggestions for how you can best protect yourself and your practice from legal action. The information in this chapter is not designed to replace the value of individualized legal or risk management consultation.

PATIENT SUICIDES AND LEGAL ACTION

Sadly, many clinicians will experience the death of a client or patient by suicide. Data suggest that 50% of psychiatrists (Chemtob, Hamada, Bauer, Kinney, & Torigoe, 1988; Ruskin, Sakinofsky, Bagby, Dickens, & Sousa, 2004) and 20% of psychologists (Chemtob, Hamada, Bauer, Torigoe, & Kinney, 1988) will have a patient die by suicide at some point during their careers. Approximately one in nine psychology interns/trainees will have a patient die by suicide, and another one in four interns/trainees will have a client make a suicide attempt (Kleespies, Penk, & Forsyth, 1993). Obviously, not all clinicians are sued following a client suicide. Among those clinicians who do have legal action taken against them, few end up going to trial. As few as 6% of these cases end up in court, and most of them are won by clinicians (Packman & Harris, 1998).

For those clinicians who do find themselves involved in a legal action, the experience can be stressful for many reasons. In addition to the grief reactions shared by most suicide survivors, treating clinicians faced with legal action are placed in the vulnerable and uncomfortable position of having their professional care of a patient scrutinized by the legal system. The best strategy to protect oneself legally is a preventive approach: knowing the law, the standard of care, and how best to document your care. The concept of "therapeutic risk management" is important (Simon & Shuman, 2009). This refers to successfully managing clinical–legal dilemmas while maintaining a focus on the quality of the client or patient's clinical care.

What Is Malpractice?

Malpractice complaints fall under what is called tort law. A tort is a civil wrong (not criminal). This wrongful act can be an intentional or negligent act that involves an injury/damage to another.

Malpractice is the failure to assess or treat a patient in compliance with the applicable standard of care resulting in injury or damage. The applicable standard of care is defined by what the average, reasonable, and prudent clinician would do when faced with the same or similar circumstances, as opined by experts. A breach occurs when a clinician fails to provide care consistent with the standard of care and that breach results in injury or damage. It does not matter if the breach in the standard of care was unintentional (Simon, 2001).

While anyone can file a lawsuit, to prove malpractice, one must substantiate a viable "cause of action." To do this, a medical malpractice plaintiff must establish four elements:

1. Duty of care (established clinician–patient relationship).
2. Breach of the standard of care.
3. Injury/harm to the patient.
4. Injury must be proximately caused by and in proximity to the professional's substandard conduct.

These four elements for malpractice are commonly summarized by the "four Ds": Dereliction of Duty Directly causing Damages (Rachlin, 1984).

Whether the medical malpractice plaintiff has proven the four elements is determined by the trier of fact (a judge or a jury). While malpractice cases can be tried with a ruling by a judge, most often they are tried in front of a jury. Should a malpractice suit be tried in court, it is done in a civil court held to the standard, in most states, of "preponderance of evidence." Preponderance of evidence refers to the greater weight of evidence for one side. It is based on more convincing evidence and probable truth and accuracy, and not solely based on the actual *amount* of evidence.

What Should a Clinician Do If He or She Is Named in a Lawsuit?

If you are named in a lawsuit or threatened with legal action, the first action you should take is to contact your attorney, your agency's risk management department, and/or your malpractice insurance carrier. Many hospitals will have attorneys on staff. If you are in private practice, you may want to consider hiring an attorney with expertise in medical malpractice. Although you may be represented by an attorney who works for your malpractice insurance company, involving a personal attorney will also assure that your individual interests are protected. Do not discuss the patient or the family's claims with anyone before you speak with your attorney, risk manager, or malpractice carrier. Good legal counsel should direct you on the best course of action.

What Are the Malpractice Issues Related to Suicide?

Clinicians are held to a standard of care related to the proper assessment and management of suicidal patients (e.g., Berman, 2006; Simon, 2002). There are two central issues that are a common source of legal pitfalls in cases regarding a patient death by suicide.

The first issue or potential legal pitfall is that of *foreseeability*—did the clinician appropriately assess for suicide? To avoid malpractice, a suicide risk assessment based on available sources of information must be conducted (see Chapter 4). These sources are often multiple and sometimes require extra efforts for us to elicit (e.g., asking appropriate questions, using collateral sources, or obtaining medical records).

The second legal pitfall is *causation*. Did the clinician do something (or, more commonly, neglect to do something) that may have caused the suicide? Once suicide risk is identified, we need to respond with reasonable efforts to protect the patient from harm (Vandecreek, Knapp, & Herzog, 1987). Our response should involve building and implementing a comprehensive treatment plan (Berman, Jobes, & Silverman, 2006) based on good clinical practice (see Chapter 5).

What Can Clinicians Do to Protect Themselves from Liability?

No measures can protect you entirely from having a lawsuit filed. When a death by suicide occurs, family members grieve and may look for someone to blame as a way to cope with the tragic event. As a clinician working with high-risk teens, there are ways of protecting oneself from litigation.

A first way is to form a strong alliance with the teen's family. Keep the family informed of the teen's suicide risk factors, progress in treatment, and what you are doing to reduce the risk. Open communication with the family about what you can and cannot do is important. For instance, telling the parents that you will do everything you can to help their child, but that you cannot control his or her behavior outside of your office, and that treatment will take time are all important aspects to forming this alliance.

Legal case law (reviewed by Bongar et al., 1998) also provides us with suggestions for key areas to include in your assessment and treatment that may be helpful to minimize liability. However, this list is not meant to be all inclusive. You should always practice appropriate care based on the specific facts of each case. Earlier chapters in this book provide information about risk factors, comprehensive risk assessment and formulation, and the importance of strong documentation.

Minimizing Liability

- Obtain a thorough history.
  - o Gather sufficient detail from the patient.
  - o Utilize collateral sources of information.
  - o Obtain medical records or information from previous clinicians.
- Assess for suicide risk.
  - o Risk assessment should be done at first visit, critical points in treatment, and at regular intervals throughout treatment.
  - o Use evidence-based practices to stratify the level of risk.
- Follow the standard of care.
  - o The standard of care should be followed as closely as possible.
  - o If the clinical facts indicate deviating from the standard of care, you should document these reasons carefully and consider a second opinion.
- Evaluate for and respond to suicidal intent.

- Be available with backup and emergency coverage.
  - Be available during reasonable hours.
  - Let patients know how to access help if you are not immediately available (e.g., the local emergency department or crisis phone numbers).
- Increase frequency of visits for high-risk individuals and/or consider follow-up phone calls.
- Involve family and friends in care.
  - Communicate information about a minor's suicide intent to his or her parents.
- Involve family in assessment, treatment planning, and care.
  - Obtain supervision and/or consultation (second opinion) for high-risk cases.
  - Document clearly, in a timely manner, and carefully.
- Treat the patient in the most appropriate setting.
  - Recommend inpatient care or commit patients when necessary (depends on state laws).
  - Discharge from the inpatient setting only when clinically appropriate.
- Utilize appropriate suicide precautions.
  - In the inpatient setting: seclusion, restraints, increased supervision, locked unit.
  - Remove dangerous objects (e.g., contraband in the inpatient setting) and recommend firearm removal or other potential dangers in outpatient care.
- Use medications properly.
  - Refer for a medication assessment when indicated.
  - If prescribing medications, use the appropriate doses and monitoring.

As presented in Chapter 5, good and thorough documentation is an essential aid in your defense. You can provide the best clinical care but still be at risk for litigation, particularly if your assessment and treatment are not appropriately documented. From a legal perspective, if something wasn't written down, it didn't happen (Gutheil, 1980). It is therefore critical to write thorough and accurate clinical notes in a timely fashion.

When documenting, explain why you chose one decision over another. An effective way of doing so is to articulate your thoughts or rationale on paper. Gutheil (1980) explains this as "thinking out loud for the record." In this process, you can put your reasons for and against a particular decision to show that you have weighed foreseeable risks and benefits to come to a reasonable conclusion.

What Are Other Essential Elements of the Clinical Record?

Any informed consent needed for treatment should be documented. Some jurisdictions require written informed consent for mental health care. If written consent is obtained, you should certainly include it as a part of the medical record. However, written consent is only one component of informed consent. Informed consent can be thought of as a process or ongoing conversation about the indications, risks, benefits, and alternatives to treatment. Documenting that this conversation took place and any questions that came up can be more helpful than simply obtaining a signature.

Communications with family or phone calls should also be documented. Conversations with families about suicide risk should be considered akin to informed consent about medication and shouldn't be missed in your documentation.

Should you obtain a second opinion or get clinical supervision on a case, it is also helpful to include acknowledgment of these elements in your medical record. An actual copy of the second opinion can be added to your record.

Issues of Confidentiality: Beyond Therapeutic Principles

Involving family and friends and communicating with other care providers can be essential to the safe and effective treatment of suicidal patients, but it is important that we are knowledgeable about our legal responsibilities with respect to confidential health information. The Health Insurance Portability and Accountability Act (HIPAA) is a federal act that was enacted in 1996, and later modified in August of 2002. HIPAA protects all "individually identifiable health information" in any form or media. It gives patients an array of rights with respect to that information. One of these rights is to protect the release of health information to family or friends. Under this legislation, a medical professional can only release protected health information if he or she has permission from the patient or the patient's personal representative.

How Do Confidentiality Laws Address Minors?

For minors, the personal representative is most often the parent or guardian. In this case, the parent or guardian would have rights to the protected health information of his or her child. Although HIPAA is a federal law applicable to all 50 states and the District of Columbia, it is actually subordinate to state law. Therefore, state laws, where in existence, may create exceptions to the parents' or guardians' rights to the health care information about their minor children. Twenty states and the District of Columbia have such laws. In these areas, minors are given explicit authority to consent to outpatient mental health services. In some of these states, there is a minimum age for this exception, and in some the clinician maintains the authority to notify the parents (Boonstra & Nash, 2000). Essentially, in many of these states, a minor has the right to disclose or withhold protected health information from his or her parents.

HIPAA also specifies what to do if there is no state law with which to defer. If the state law is silent concerning parental access to the minor's protected health information, a clinician has discretion to provide or deny a parent access to the minor's health information, provided the decision is made by a licensed health care professional in the exercise of professional judgment. It is important that you know your state's legal regulations with respect to minors and their protected health care information.

When Should I "Breach" Confidentiality?

Unfortunately, there is no clear legal direction as to when we can "breach" confidentiality. Court decisions have not been consistent with respect to confidentiality in mental health practice involving safety issues. The well-known Tarasoff case (Vitaly Tarasoff et al. v. The Regents of the University of California et al.) ruled that one has a duty to protect an identified intended victim. Some may argue that the identified victim may be the person himself in the case of suicide, thereby permitting or even indicating that a clinician should involve family or friends if deemed to be helpful in managing safety risk. However, a later court case was not consistent with this line of thinking. This court case in 1978 (Melanie Bellah et al. v. Daniel P. Greenson) ruled that the patient's confidentiality outweighs the societal interest of informing family members of a patient's suicide potential.

Although legal rulings have not provided a clear guide to confidentiality issues for suicidal patients, there are some clinical approaches that we find helpful. As mentioned in the confidentiality section of this book (Chapter 5), setting the stage is essential. Communicating guidelines with each patient (and parents, as appropriate) at the beginning of treatment sets the stage for how we might handle an acute safety concern, should one arise in the treatment process. The clinician should share his or her policy on safety concerns and confidentiality and have the patient and parents agree about a person to whom safety concerns would be communicated. If a patient is thought to be a serious threat to his or her own health or the safety of others, one can then consider making a disclosure according to the already agreed-upon guidelines. This disclosure should be made to a person whom they believe can prevent or lessen the threat. Careful documentation is essential to minimize potential legal consequences in this process. It is also important that all clinicians be familiar with and adhere to their state's laws. In addition, a collaborative care approach, as described in Chapters 5 and 6, may lessen legal risk. Parents who sue are often angry and are reacting to feeling disenfranchised in some way from their child's treatment team. Parents who have been well informed and who have felt they are part of the treatment process from the beginning are unlikely to pursue legal action, even after a tragic event.

CONCLUSION

Many teens at elevated risk for suicide are either effectively treated or "recover" sufficiently to function reasonably well at home, in school, and with friends. Nevertheless, working with these at-risk teens can evoke fears among clinicians, such as fear of a tragic outcome and/or fear of a potential lawsuit. Fortunately, the fear of a potential lawsuit is much more prevalent than the risk of ending up in a courtroom. This chapter provides information about legal risk in addition to suggestions about how clinicians can protect themselves from legal action. The information is not designed to replace the value of individualized legal or risk management consultation.

Appendix

Risk Factor Checklist
for Teen Suicidal Behavior and Suicide

Demographic Characteristics

- Gender
  - ◆ Male (suicide)
  - ◆ Female (nonfatal suicidal behavior)
- Racial and ethnic background
  - ◆ Black females have lowest suicide rate
  - ◆ Native American/Alaskan Native males have highest suicide rate

Clinical Features

- Previous suicide attempt
  - ◆ Multiple previous attempts (two or more) = highest risk
- Suicidal ideation and/or intent
  - ◆ Especially plans and preparation
- Psychiatric disorders
  - ◆ Depressive or bipolar disorder
  - ◆ Alcohol/drug abuse
  - ◆ Conduct disorder
  - ◆ Posttraumatic stress disorder
  - ◆ Other (e.g., anxiety disorder, schizophrenia, eating disorder)
- Other behaviors and characteristics
  - ◆ Nonsuicidal self-injury
  - ◆ Hopelessness
  - ◆ Impulsivity
  - ◆ Psychic pain
  - ◆ Poor reality testing
  - ◆ Aggressive tendencies or history of violent behavior
  - ◆ Cluster B and C traits
  - ◆ Personality disorder
  - ◆ Sleep disturbance/insomnia
  - ◆ Learning disorders and difficulties
- Recent discharge from psychiatric hospital; recent change in treatment

Family and Interpersonal Factors

- Family history of suicidal behaviors, suicide
- Family history of psychiatric disorder
- Sexual abuse, physical abuse
- Bullying victimization and/or perpetration
- Peer relationship difficulties, poor social integration
- Family conflict, low support, perceived burdensomeness
- Lesbian, gay, bisexual, transgender

Contextual Factors

- Exposure to suicide
- Access to lethal means (firearm)

Recent Life Stress

- Loss of/conflict in close relationship
- Disciplinary action, shame experience

Tracking Form for School-Based Screening

Student Name	Date of Positive Screen	Date of Follow-Up	Date Parents Notified	Referral/ Recommendation	Date of Follow-Up to Assess Service Utilization

Suicide Prevention Resources for Schools
(Guidelines and Education/Awareness Programs)

Program	Description
Curriculum-based education/awareness programs for students	
LEADS for Youth: Linking Education and Awareness of Depression and Suicide *www.sprc.org/sites/ sprc.org/files/bpr/ LEADSBPRfactsheet.pdf*	Located on the SPRC registry for evidence-based programs, LEADS is a 3-day curriculum for high school students that teaches information about depression and suicide. Students discuss how and where to find help for themselves or depressed friends and how to overcome barriers to receiving help.
Look Listen Link *www.sprc.org/sites/sprc.org/ files/bpr/LOOKLISTENLINK. pdf*	Located on the SPRC registry for evidence-based programs, the Look Listen Link curriculum is designed for middle school–age youth. Consisting of four 45-minute sessions, it helps youth to identify causes of stress and methods for coping. Its interactive exercises empower youth to recognize signs of depression in their peers and themselves and connect them to help.
Staff inservice trainings	
AAS School Suicide Prevention Accreditation Program *www.suicidology.org/ certification-programs/ school-professionals*	This self-paced independent study training program was designed to help school districts to train a suicide prevention specialist for their community. The brief curriculum teaches warning signs, prevention and postvention principles, how to reintegrate a student after an attempt, and how to deal with a traumatic loss. The program also details the risk factors for suicide, how to assess risk, how to deal with the parents of a teen at risk, and how to create a safety contract for a student.
Making Educators Partners in Suicide Prevention (PowerPoint) *www.sptsnj.org/educators*	This 2-hour training session on suicide awareness for school personnel is a completely prepared PowerPoint presentation with notes available for no cost online. It highlights why suicide awareness training is beneficial for the entire school community. School faculty learn to correct myths about suicide and are taught accurate

(continued)

	information about suicide risk, warning signs, and protective factors. In addition, faculty learn how to interact with at-risk youth and identify helpful resources for at-risk students.
Center for Safe and Responsible Internet Use *www.embracecivility.org*	This site provides information regarding risk issues and contains a recommended action plan for intervention and prevention of cyber-bullying. The website provides free student handouts geared toward "cyber safety" for different age groups. School districts or individual teachers may purchase a 2-hour professional development presentation that gives teachers a comprehensive understanding of digital media safety and responsibility.
Schoolwide screening approaches	
SOS Signs of Suicide *www. mentalhealthscreening.org/ programs/youth-prevention-programs/sos*	A 2-day secondary school–based intervention that includes screening, education, and training. Students are screened for depression and suicide risk and referred for professional help as indicated.
Yellow Ribbon Suicide Prevention Program *www.yellowribbon.org*	The Yellow Ribbon website provides a list of programs and upcoming events and includes resources for training and education for professionals, families, and survivors. The site contains warning signs and risk factors for suicide, information and registration for gatekeeper training, and resources for depression and suicide prevention.
TeenScreen	Identifies middle school- and high school-age youth in need of mental health services due to risk for suicide and undetected mental illness. The program's main objective is to assist in the early identification of problems.
General information	
Maine Youth Suicide Prevention, Intervention, and Postvention Guidelines: A Resource for School Personnel *www.maine.gov/suicide/ docs/Guidelines%2010-2009--w%20discl.pdf*	The 63-page report examines school-based prevention for youth suicide. It highlights suicide prevention protocols in the school setting including a crisis plan, guidelines for high-risk situations, guidelines for suicide attempts in and out of school, and postvention protocols. Postvention protocols include the responsibility of school staff in the aftermath of suicide or a suicide attempt.

(continued)

155

National Association of School Psychologists. Preventing Youth Suicide: Tips for Parents and Educators *www.nasponline.org/ resources/crisis_safety/ suicideprevention.aspx*	Provides tips for educators, including suicide risk factors and warning signs. In addition, it includes what actions to take when there are signs of suicide, the role of school in suicide prevention, and resiliency factors that can lessen the potential of risk factors that lead to suicidal ideation.
The Youth Suicide Prevention School-Based Guide *theguide.fmhi.usf.edu*	This guide provides user-friendly information to evaluate school suicide prevention programs and improve on them. It defines elements of a comprehensive school-based suicide intervention program, offers successful strategies used to reduce the incidence of suicide, and provides checklists to evaluate school prevention programs. It also provides guides for school faculty to enact proven strategies for suicide prevention supported by literature and current research.
AAS Guidelines for School-Based Suicide Prevention Programs *www.sprc.org/sites/sprc. org/files/library/aasguide-school.pdf*	These guidelines examine the requirements for school-based prevention programs designed for an entire school, as well as programs designed for a selected group of at-risk students.
Stop Bullying Now Campaign *www.stopbullying.gov*	This site provides information specifically for administrators, educators, and adults at school, in addition to information tailored for children or parents. The website suggests 10 "best practice" strategies in bullying prevention and intervention, has tip sheets on how to intervene on the spot during a bullying situation, and advice on how best to support a victim of bullying.

Questions to Ask about Suicidal Thoughts

- I wonder if you've been so down that you've had thoughts about death or wishing you were dead?

- Do you ever get images or pictures in your head of your own death?

- Have you considered harming yourself? *or* How often do you feel so down that you feel like harming yourself?

- Given the severe pain you're in with this depression, and all you're dealing with at school and at home *(tailor to teen)*, I wonder if you've had thoughts of suicide?

- It sounds like you've been really down. Sometimes when teens feel so down and experience major disappointments like you have, they have thoughts of suicide. I'm wondering how often you feel so down that you have thoughts of suicide?

- Are you thinking about suicide?

- Do you sometimes have an impulse to kill yourself? How often do you have such an impulse and when (where, under what circumstances) do you have this impulse?

- How long have you been thinking about suicide? When did you first begin to have suicidal thoughts?

- How often do you have these thoughts?

- How long do the thoughts last? How hard is it to get them out of your mind?

- Have you had thoughts about how you would do it?

- What thoughts or plans do you have?

- Have you taken steps toward this plan? (The clinician may want to follow up with a more specific question; e.g., if a plan was shared to overdose: "Have you ever taken out a pill bottle?")

- Is there any part of you that wants to die?

- Do you have the intent to die?

- What stops you from doing something to harm yourself?

- What are some of the reasons you want to be living next week, next month, and next year?

Teen Suicide Risk Assessment Worksheet

Evaluator _____ **Date** _____

Client _____

Gender: M F Birthdate: _____ **Age (years):** _____

Reason for Comprehensive Risk Assessment (e.g., recent suicide attempt, reported suicidal thoughts, hospital discharge/disposition, new client, other):

_____

_____

Sources of Information (Circle):	Teen	Parent/Guardian	Other

Interview with _____

Interview with _____

Interview Form or Questionnaire (specify) _____

Other Source(s) of Information (specify)_____

Current or History of Suicidal Thoughts: **YES**   **NO**
If yes:
What is content of thoughts?

_____

Time Course (today? past week? past month? lifetime?) _____

Frequency _____

Duration (How unrelenting?) _____

Has client considered a method? _____

Does client have a plan? _____

Any preparatory action(s) _____

Are there triggers that can be identified? _____

Recent or History of Suicide Attempt: **YES**   **NO**
If yes:
How many suicide attempts? _____

(continued)

Most Recent Suicide Attempt

When (Date and Circumstances) _____

_____

Method _____

Intent (quality and level; e.g., ambivalent, fleeting, definite with advance planning) _____

_____

Possible function(s) of attempt _____

_____

Situation and triggers? _____

Previous Suicide Attempt(s)—Summarize

When (date and circumstances) _____

_____

Methods _____

Intent (quality and level; e.g., ambivalent, fleeting, definite with advance planning) _____

_____

Possible function(s) of attempts _____

Situations and triggers? _____

Other Clinical Risk Factors: Check all that apply.

☐ **Psychiatric disorder**

    ☐ Depressive/bipolar disorder

    ☐ Alcohol/drug abuse

    ☐ Conduct disorder

    ☐ Posttraumatic stress disorder

    ☐ Other

☐ **Contextual/Interpersonal**

    ☐ Social isolation

    ☐ Victim of bullying

    ☐ Lesbian/gay/bisexual/transgender

    ☐ Exposure to suicidal behavior

    ☐ Local cluster

☐ **Other Clinical**

    ☐ Previous suicide attempt

    ☐ Suicide ideation/impulses

    ☐ Poor reality testing

    ☐ Aggression/violent history

    ☐ Trauma or abuse

    ☐ Family suicide/psychiatric disorder

    ☐ Loss of close relationship

    ☐ Shame experience

    ☐ Recent psychiatric discharge

    ☐ Hopelessness

    ☐ Impulsivity

    ☐ Psychic pain

    ☐ Sleep disturbance/insomnia

    ☐ Anxiety

(continued)

Mental Status Exam: Check items present to a clinically significant degree.

☐ Psychic pain   ☐ Poor reality testing

☐ Inability to see/consider options   ☐ Depressed mood

☐ Hopelessness   ☐ Anxiety

☐ Perceived burdensomeness   ☐ Anger

☐ Shame/self-hate   ☐ Command hallucination

☐ Alcohol or drug intoxication

☐ Impulsivity

☐ Aggressive behavior

☐ Poor judgment

☐ Agitation

Notes: _____

_____

_____

Protective Factors:

Family and/or other social support (describe) _____

_____

Problem-solving/coping skills (describe) _____

_____

Future orientation and reasons for living (describe what teen is looking forward to, etc.)

_____

Cultural/religious/community beliefs (describe) _____

_____

Connectedness to others (describe) _____

_____

Risk Formulation (see Appendix F, Documentation of Teen Suicide Risk Assessment).

_____

_____

_____

_____

_____

_____

_____

_____

Documentation of Teen Suicide Risk Assessment

Evaluator _____ Assessment Date/Time _____

Client _____

Risk factors (psychiatric disorders, active use of alcohol or drugs, history of trauma/abuse/family suicide, recent stress, hospital discharge/treatment change, contextual factor such as victimization/bullying):

_____

_____

Suicidal thoughts, impulses; history of suicide attempts (Thoughts: content, severity, frequency, controllability; Attempts: number, precipitants, method, functional analysis):

_____

_____

Mental status (current psychological functioning):

_____

_____

Protective Factors:

_____

_____

Risk formulation (summarize risk and protective factors; indicate judgment regarding level of risk):

_____

_____

_____

_____

Plan of action:

_____

_____

_____

_____

SAFE-T Card

SAFE-T

Suicide **A**ssessment **F**ive-step
Evaluation and **T**riage

for Mental Health Professionals

1 IDENTIFY RISK FACTORS
Note those that can be modified to reduce risk

2 IDENTIFY PROTECTIVE FACTORS
Note those that can be enhanced

3 CONDUCT SUICIDE INQUIRY
Suicidal thoughts, plans behavior and intent

4 DETERMINE RISK LEVEL/INTERVENTION
Determine risk. Choose appropriate intervention to address and reduce risk

5 DOCUMENT
Assessment of risk, rationale, intervention and follow-up

NATIONAL SUICIDE PREVENTION LIFELINE
1.800.273.TALK (8255)

RESOURCES

- Download this card and additional resources at
  www.sprc.org or at www.stopasuicide.org
- Resource for implementing The Joint Commission 2007
  Patient Safety Goals on Suicide
  www.sprc.org/library/jcsafetygoals.pdf
- SAFE-T drew upon the American Psychiatric Association
  Practice Guidelines for the Assessment and Treatment of
  Patients with Suicidal Behaviors www.psychiatryonline.
  com/pracGuide/pracGuideTopic_14.aspx
- Practice Parameter for the Assessment and Treatment of
  Children and Adolescents with Suicidal Behavior. Journal
  of the American Academy of Child and Adolescent
  Psychiatry, 2001, 40 (7 Supplement): 24s-51s

ACKNOWLEDGEMENTS

- Originally conceived by Douglas Jacobs, MD, and developed
  as a collaboration between Screening for Mental Health,
  Inc. and the Suicide Prevention Resource Center.
- This material is based upon work supported by the
  Substance Abuse and Mental Health Services Administration
  (SAMHSA) under Grant No. 1U79SM57392. Any opinions/
  findings/conclusions/recommendations expressed in this
  material are those of the author and do not necessarily
  reflect the views of SAMHSA.

National Suicide Prevention Lifeline
1.800.273.TALK (8255)

www.sprc.org   www.mentalhealthscreening.org

Suicide assessments should be conducted at first contact, with any subsequent suicidal behavior, increased ideation, or pertinent clinical change; for inpatients, prior to increasing privileges and at discharge.

1. RISK FACTORS

✓ **Suicidal behavior:** history of prior suicide attempts, aborted suicide attempts or self-injurious behavior
✓ **Current/past psychiatric disorders:** especially mood disorders, psychotic disorders, alcohol/substance abuse, ADHD, TBI, PTSD, Cluster B personality disorders, conduct disorders (antisocial behavior, aggression, impulsivity).
  Co-morbidity and recent onset of illness increase risk
✓ **Key symptoms:** anhedonia, impulsivity, hopelessness, anxiety/panic, insomnia, command hallucinations
✓ **Family history:** of suicide, attempts or Axis 1 psychiatric disorders requiring hospitalization
✓ **Precipitants/Stressors/Interpersonal:** triggering events leading to humiliation, shame or despair (e.g., loss of relationship, financial or health status--real or anticipated). Ongoing medical illness (esp. CNS disorders, pain). Intoxication. Family turmoil/chaos. History of physical or sexual abuse. Social isolation.
✓ **Change in treatment:** discharge from psychiatric hospital, provider or treatment change
✓ **Access to firearms**

2. PROTECTIVE FACTORS *Protective factors, even if present, may not counteract significant acute risk*

✓ **Internal:** ability to cope with stress, religious beliefs, frustration tolerance
✓ **External:** responsibility to children or beloved pets, positive therapeutic relationships, social supports

3. SUICIDE INQUIRY *Specific questioning about thoughts, plans, behaviors, intent*

✓ **Ideation:** frequency, intensity, duration--in last 48 hours, past month and worst ever
✓ **Plan:** timing, location, lethality, availability, preparatory acts
✓ **Behaviors:** past attempts, aborted attempts, rehearsals (tying noose, loading gun), vs. non-suicidal self injurious actions
✓ **Intent:** extent to which the patient (1) expects to carry out the plan and (2) believes the plan/act to be lethal vs. self-injurious;
  Explore ambivalence: reasons to die vs. reasons to live

° For Youths: ask parent/ guardian about evidence of suicidal thoughts, plans, or behaviors, and changes in mood, behaviors or disposition
° Homicide Inquiry: when indicated, esp. in character disordered or paranoid males dealing with loss or humiliation. Inquire in four areas listed above.

4. RISK LEVEL/INTERVENTION

✓ Assessment of risk level is based on clinical judgment, after completing steps 1-3
✓ Reassess as patient or environmental circumstances change

RISK LEVEL	RISK / PROTECTIVE FACTOR	SUICIDALITY	POSSIBLE INTERVENTIONS
High	Psychiatric disorders with severe symptoms, or acute precipitating event; protective factors not relevant	Potentially (lethal suicide attempt or persistent ideation with strong intent or suicide rehearsal	Admission generally indicated unless a significant change reduces risk. Suicide precautions
Moderate	Multiple risk factors, few protective factors	Suicidal ideation with plan, but no intent or behavior	Admission may be necessary depending on risk factors. Develop crisis plan. Give emergency/crisis numbers
Low	Modifiable risk factors, strong protective factors	Thoughts of death, no plan, intent or behavior	Outpatient referral, symptom reduction. Give emergency/crisis numbers

(This chart is intended to represent a range of risk levels and interventions, not actual determinations.)

5. DOCUMENT

Risk level and rationale; treatment plan to address/reduce current risk (e.g., setting, medication, psychotherapy, E.C.T., contact with significant others, consultation); firearm instructions, if relevant; follow up plan. For youths, treatment plan should include roles for parent/guardian.

163

Safety Plan Form

1. What are my triggers for suicidal thoughts or self-harmful behaviors? How might I recognize when I need to take steps to protect my well-being and remain safe?

_____

_____

2. The steps I will take when I experience these triggers, suicidal thoughts, or self-harm urges:

   a. Try to relax by _____

   b. Do something physically active such as _____

   c. Distract myself by _____

   d. Use coping statements (thoughts) such as _____

   _____

   _____

   e. Contact a family member, friend, support person:

   Name   Phone Number

   _____   _____

   _____   _____

   _____   _____

   _____   _____

   _____   _____

   f. Call my therapist or emergency numbers OR go to emergency department:

   Emergency: 911

   Local emergency services: _____

   My clinical provider/therapist: _____

   (Times I can reach my clinical provider) _____

   Suicide Prevention Lifeline: 1-800-273-TALK (8255)

   g. Move away from any method or means for hurting myself; involve family member or support person in limiting my access to means.

   (continued)

---

3. A couple of things that are very important to me and worth living for are:

_____

_____

Signed:

_____
Client   Date

_____
Therapist   Date

_____
Parent/Guardian (if possible)   Date

Suicide Warning Signs for Parents

Be aware that the following factors may be a warning or risk for suicide:

- Depression and other mental health disorders.
- Noticeable change in behavior, high anxiety, or agitation.
- Talking, writing, or communicating about suicide or death.
- Inability to sleep.
- Buying a gun.
- Past suicide attempts or suicidal behaviors.
- Substance use (drugs and alcohol).
- Hearing about someone else's suicide.

Precautions to take:

- Remove all weapons, including firearms, from the home.
- Lock up prescription and over-the-counter medications.
- Monitor your teen's behavior more closely.
- Ask your teen daily about his/her mood and for the presence of suicidal thoughts.
- Screen contacts with problematic peers or others.

What to do if your teen feels suicidal:

- Work with your teen on his/her safety plan.
- Contact his/her therapist or psychiatrist.
- Call a crisis number (national crisis hotline: 1-800-273-8255).
- Go to the emergency department.
- Call 911.

Tips for Communicating with Teens

1. **Be genuine**. It is better to say less to a teenager than to try and say things that one does not genuinely believe.

2. **Convey warmth and openness**. Convey warmth, caring, and a willingness to hear youth speak about a variety of topics. Some of these topics may make us uncomfortable. The idea is to "hear the youth out" rather than to "stop them in their tracks" with an interruption, comment that we don't agree, or statement like "Everything will be fine" or "I don't think it's so bad."

3. **Listen carefully and make an effort to understand the teen's perspective**. It may be helpful to consider the following steps:

   a. Rephrase and clarify what the teen said. Perhaps repeat it in your own words to check out whether you understood correctly what the teen was saying.

   b. Acknowledge the teen's thoughts and feelings. It is not necessary to agree with the teen's thoughts and feelings, but it is helpful to recognize them.

   c. Offer your own feelings and thoughts on the matter. The best time to do this is after you have listened carefully and acknowledged the teen's perspective.

4. **Use "I" statements**. These would include sentences such as, "I like the way you handled that situation," or "I am concerned about what you're saying happened." These kinds of statements convey a personal and genuine interest. They are preferred over statements like, "You make me upset," or "You handled that the way you usually do."

5. **Use specific statements when giving feedback**. That is, say something like "I think it's great that you earned a B in algebra," rather than "You're a great student." Or "I think you made a mistake by drinking with Roy last night," rather than "You're a drunk and can't seem to change." Whenever possible, avoid vague, general feedback statements that can hurt, increase hopelessness, and leave too much room for misunderstanding.

6. **Obtain input from the youth about how you can best support him or her**. For example, let the teen guide you about the best times to check in about his/her mood or how things are going at school or with friends. Provide the teen with some choices in how to structure the nature of your support. For example, "How do you feel about me reminding you to take your medicine? I could just leave it out for you in the mornings, I could leave you a note or text you to remind you, or I could verbally remind you before you leave for school. What makes you most comfortable?"

Useful Websites

Website	Unique Features
www.sprc.org Suicide Prevention Resource Center The SPRC website contains valuable resources, such as a best practices registry and a toolkit for suicide prevention for primary care providers. The site also provides information for online training workshops as well as a history of suicide prevention activities in the United States. SPRC also sends a free weekly e-mail newsletter with updates from the field of suicide prevention.	• Customized information for people in many different roles regarding suicide risks and warning signs. • Access to SPRC prevention specialists. • Best practice information regarding suicide prevention, including gatekeeper training. • Online library of resources.
www.suicidepreventionlifeline.com National Suicide Prevention Lifeline (1-800-273-TALK)	• Information about the national suicide prevention crisis line. • The lifeline gallery, real stories of hope and recovery added by survivors.
www.nimh.nih.gov/health/topics/suicide-prevention/index.shtml National Institute of Mental Health The NIMH website contains information on recent research in the field of mental health, broadcasts opportunities for public involvement, and provides substantial information about mental health problems and effective treatments.	• Risk factors for suicide. • Statistics on suicide prevalence. • Fact sheet on treatment and prevention.
www.suicidology.org American Association of Suicidology The AAS website includes information and support for researchers, suicide survivors, clinicians, and even those contemplating suicide. The site provides information regarding trainings, certifications, and recent research on suicide.	• Warning signs and risk factors for suicide. • Fact sheets regarding suicide prevalence by race/age. • Ways to become involved in suicide prevention. • Annual suicide prevention conference.

(continued)

www.afsp.org American Foundation for Suicide Prevention The AFSP site outlines prevention projects and provides educational resources. There are opportunities to join an AFSP chapter and information for suicide prevention researchers seeking grant funding.	• Warning signs and risk factors for suicide. • Facts and figures for different ages, races, and special populations. • Information on what to do when you suspect someone is considering suicide. • Opportunities to get involved in suicide prevention at a local level.
www.mentalhealthamerica.net Mental Health America This website contains information on a variety of mental health disorders, treatments, and topics. It provides resources for finding treatment and support groups.	• Wide range of mental health topics. • Different treatments that may help someone who is considering suicide. • Can search on "suicide" for information on suicide warning signs, helping someone at risk, and resources.
www.effectivechildtherapy.com Association of Behavioral and Cognitive Therapies Society for Clinical Child and Adolescent Psychology The joint website between the ABCT and SCCAP provides up-to-date information on the best treatments available for a wide variety of mental health problems. It contains a directory for the general public to find therapists and offers information for clinicians on empirically supported treatments.	• Available sources for treatment. • Information on the best treatment practices for specific problems. • Online function to search for therapists in specific fields, including suicide and adolescents.
www.mentalhealthscreening.org Screening for Mental Health The Screening for Mental Health website offers information on mental health screening for a variety of settings, including military, community, schools, workplace, and health care.	• Fact sheets on suicide and depression. • Screening and online kits (fee). • Sample online screenings for a variety of mental health problems.

(continued)

www.yspp.org Washington State Youth Suicide Prevention Program The Washington State Youth Suicide Prevention Program website provides a great deal of information for schools, parents, and youth. The website has a large list of available resources broken down into different regions of the state.	• A list of frequently asked questions regarding risk factors and warning signs. • Specific information and resources for GLBTQ youth. • Information regarding available training sessions in suicide prevention programs.
www.reachout.com A website meant for teens developed by SAMHSA and the Ad Council with teen input. Education is provided about suicide and other risk factors. Teens share stories via videos and blogs; resources are provided to help teens help one another.	• Educational resources designed for teens. • Teens submit their personal stories of struggle and recovery. • Resources are provided for teens to help a friend and get involved in their community prevention activities.
www.hsph.harvard.edu/means-matter Harvard Injury Control Research Center (part of Harvard School of Public Health) The Means Matter Campaign website contains many statistics and resources regarding the question of *how* people are taking their lives, as opposed to simply *why*. The site provides information about the importance of means reduction in suicide prevention.	• Frequently asked questions regarding the effects of means reduction on suicide. • A free online course on means reduction. • A "means matters" slide show that can be used to spread the word about lethal means reduction.
www.cdc.gov/violenceprevention/pub/selfdirected_ violence.html This website contains free access and information regarding the Self-Directed Violence Surveillance: Uniform Definitions and Recommended Data Elements report.	• Report provides background information on self-directed violence and its importance. • Outlines uniform definitions of self-directed violence. • Recommends data elements for use with collection of suicide information.

Evidence-Based
Youth Suicide Interventions

See the Substance Abuse and Mental Health Services Administration's National Registry of Evidence-Based Programs and Practices website (*www.nrepp.samhsa.gov*).

Intervention	Description
Education and training	
American Indian Life Skills Development/ Zuni Life Skills Development	A school-based suicide prevention curriculum designed to reduce suicide risk and improve protective factors among American Indian adolescents 14–19 years old.
CARE (Care, Assess, Respond, Empower)	Formerly called Counselors CARE (C-CARE) and Measure of Adolescent Potential for Suicide (MAPS), a high school–based suicide prevention program targeting high-risk youth.
CAST (Coping And Support Training)	A high school–based suicide prevention program targeting youth 14–19 years old. CAST delivers life-skills training and social support in a small-group format (6–8 students per group).
Emergency Department Means Restriction Education	An intervention for the adult caregivers of youth (ages 6–19 years) who are seen in an emergency department and determined through a mental health assessment to be at risk for suicide.
Emergency Room Intervention for Adolescent Females	A program for girls 12–18 years old who are admitted to the emergency room after attempting suicide. The intervention, which involves the girl and one or more family members who accompany her to the emergency room, aims to increase attendance in outpatient treatment following discharge from the emergency room and to reduce future suicide attempts.
LEADS: For Youth (Linking Education and Awareness of Depression and Suicide)	A curriculum for high school students in grades 9–12 that is designed to increase knowledge of depression and suicide, modify perceptions of depression and suicide, increase knowledge of suicide prevention resources, and improve intentions to engage in help-seeking behaviors.

(continued)

Intervention	Description
Lifelines Curriculum	A comprehensive, schoolwide suicide prevention program for middle and high school students. The goal of Lifelines is to promote a caring, competent school community in which help seeking is encouraged and modeled, and suicidal behavior is recognized as an issue that cannot be kept secret.
Model Adolescent Suicide Prevention Program (MASPP)	A public health-oriented suicidal-behavior prevention and intervention program originally developed for a small American Indian tribe in rural New Mexico to target high rates of suicide among its adolescents and young adults.
QPR Gatekeeper Training for Suicide Prevention	A brief, 1–2 hour, educational program designed to teach "gatekeepers"—those who are strategically positioned to recognize and refer someone at risk of suicide (e.g., parents, friends, neighbors, teachers, coaches, caseworkers, police officers)—the warning signs of a suicide crisis and how to respond.
Reconnecting Youth: A Peer Group Approach to Building Life Skills	A school-based prevention program for students (ages 14–19 years) that teaches skills to build resiliency against risk factors and control early signs of substance abuse and emotional distress.
SOS Signs of Suicide	A 2-day secondary school-based intervention that includes screening and education. Students are screened for depression and suicide risk and referred for professional help as indicated.
Sources of Strength	A universal suicide prevention program designed to build socioecological protective influences among youth to reduce the likelihood that vulnerable high school students will become suicidal.
TeenScreen	Identifies middle school- and high school-age youth in need of mental health services due to risk for suicide and undetected mental illness. The program's main objective is to assist in the early identification of problems that might not otherwise come to the attention of professionals.
United States Air Force Suicide Prevention Program	A population-oriented approach to reducing the risk of suicide. The Air Force has implemented 11 initiatives aimed at strengthening social support, promoting development of social skills, and changing policies and norms to encourage effective help-seeking behaviors.

(continued)

Intervention	Description
Psychotherapy	
Adolescent Coping with Depression (CWD-A)	A cognitive-behavioral group intervention that targets specific problems typically experienced by depressed adolescents. These problems include discomfort and anxiety, irrational/negative thoughts, poor social skills, and limited experiences of pleasant activities.
Dialectical Behavior Therapy	A cognitive-behavioral treatment approach with two key characteristics: a behavioral, problem-solving focus blended with acceptance-based strategies and an emphasis on dialectical processes.
Multisystemic Therapy With Psychiatric Supports (MST-Psychiatric)	Designed to treat youth who are at risk for out-of-home placement (in some cases, psychiatric hospitalization) due to serious behavioral problems and co-occurring mental health symptoms such as thought disorder, bipolar affective disorder, depression, anxiety, and impulsivity.

Sample Letter to Formally Request School-Based Services

When requesting a formal evaluation, individualized education plan, or accommodations for a teen at school, parents must submit a written request to the school. According to the Individuals With Disabilities Education Act (2004), schools have 10 business days to respond to the written request and 30 business days, to complete the evaluation.

Dear (*principal, special education coordinator, resource teacher, or school mental health professional*),

My child, (*name, date of birth*), was recently evaluated at (*name of hospital or clinic*) because of concerns about (*list diagnoses or symptoms here*). The (*psychiatrist, psychologist, social worker, etc.*) has diagnosed (*him/her*) with (*list diagnoses here*). I have attached a copy of the evaluation to this letter.

We are very concerned about the impact of (*diagnosis*) on (*student's*) academic (*and/ or social, emotional, behavioral*) functioning at school. For this reason, we are formally requesting an evaluation in order to determine whether (*student's name*) would benefit from additional accommodations or services during the school day.

We hope to establish a strong partnership between our family, (*student's*) teachers, and our treatment team at (*location*) so that we can all work effectively together to help (*student*) through this difficult time.

Please contact me at (*list phone number*) to set up a time to discuss this written request for evaluation and services.

Sincerely,

(*Parent name and contact information*)

References

Achenbach, T. M., McConaughy, S. H., & Howell, C. T. (1987). Child/adolescent behavioral and emotional problems: Implications of cross-informant correlations for situational specificity. *Psychological Bulletin, 101*(2), 213–232.

Agerbo, E., Nordentoft, M., & Mortensen, P. B. (2002). Familial, psychiatric, and socioeconomic risk factors for suicide in young people: Nested case–control study. *BMJ: British Medical Journal, 325*(7355), 74–77.

American Academy of Child and Adolescent Psychiatry. (1998). Practice parameters for the assessment and treatment of children and adolescents with depressive disorders. *Journal of the American Academy of Child and Adolescent Psychiatry, 37*(Suppl.), 63S–83S.

American Academy of Child and Adolescent Psychiatry. (2001). Practice parameters for the assessment and treatment of children and adolescents with suicidal behavior. *Journal of the American Academy of Child and Adolescent Psychiatry, 40*(Suppl.), 24S–51S.

American Academy of Child and Adolescent Psychiatry. (2009). Improving mental health services in primary care: Reducing administrative and financial barriers to access and collaboration. *Pediatrics, 123*(4), 1248–1251.

American Medical Association. (2012). JAMAevidence Glossary. Retrieved May 16, 2012, from *http://jamaevidence.com/glossary*.

American Psychiatric Association. (2000). *Diagnostic and statistical manual of mental disorders* (4th ed, text rev.). Washington, DC: Author.

American Psychiatric Association. (2003). Practice guideline for the assessment and treatment of patients with suicidal behaviors.(Erratum appears in American Journal of Psychiatry (2004), *161*(4), 776). *American Journal of Psychiatry, 160*(11 Suppl.), 1–60.

American Psychiatric Association. (2006). *American Psychiatric Association practice guidelines for the treatment of psychiatric disorders: Compendium 2006.* Washington, DC: Author.

Andrews, J. A., & Lewinsohn, P. M. (1992). Suicidal attempts among older adolescents: Prevalence and co-occurrence with psychiatric disorders. *Journal of the American Academy of Child and Adolescent Psychiatry, 31*(4), 655–662.

APA Presidential Task Force on Evidence-Based Practice. (2006). Evidence-based practice in psychology. *American Psychologist, 61*(4), 271–285.

Arata, C. M., Langhinrichsen-Rohling, J., Bowers, D., & O'Brien, N. (2007). Differential correlates of multi-type maltreatment among urban youth. *Child Abuse and Neglect, 31*(4), 393–415.

Asarnow, J. R., Carlson, G. A., & Guthrie, D. (1987). Coping strategies, self-perceptions, hopelessness, and perceived family environments in depressed and suicidal children. *Journal of Consulting and Clinical Psychology, 55*(3), 361–366.

Asarnow, J. R., Porta, G., Spirito, A., Emslie, G., Clarke, G., Wagner, K. D., et al. (2011). Suicide attempts and nonsuicidal self-injury in the treatment of resistant depression in adolescents: Findings from the TORDIA study. *Journal of the American Academy of Child and Adolescent Psychiatry, 50*(8), 772–781.

Aseltine, R. H., Jr. (2003). An evaluation of a school-based suicide prevention program. *Adolescent and Family Health, 3*(2), 81–88.

Aseltine, R. H., Jr., & DeMartino, R. (2004). An outcome evaluation of the SOS suicide prevention program. *American Journal of Public Health, 94*(3), 446–451.

Aseltine, R. H., Jr., James, A., Schilling, E., & Glanovsky, J. (2007). Evaluating the SOS suicide prevention program: A replication and extension. *BMC Public Health, 7*(1), 161.

Baerger, D. R. (2001). Risk management with the suicidal patient: Lessons from case law. *Professional Psychology: Research and Practice, 32*(4), 359–366.

Baldry, A. C., & Winkel, F. W. (2003). Direct and vicarious victimization at school and at home as risk factors for suicidal cognition among Italian adolescents. *Journal of Adolescence, 26*(6), 703–716.

Barrett, P. M., Dadds, M. R., & Rapee, R. M. (1996). Family treatment of childhood anxiety: A controlled trial. *Journal of Consulting and Clinical Psychology, 64*(2), 333–342.

Beautrais, A. L., Joyce, P. R., & Mulder, R. T. (1996). Risk factors for serious suicide attempts among youths aged 13 through 24 years. *Journal of the American Academy of Child and Adolescent Psychiatry, 35*(9), 1174–1182.

Beautrais, A. L., Joyce, P. R., Mulder, R. T., & Fergusson, D. M. (1996). Prevalence and comorbidity of mental disorders in persons making serious suicide attempts: A case–control study. *American Journal of Psychiatry, 153*(8), 1009–1014.

Beck, A. T., & Steer, R. A. (1988). *Beck Hopelessness Scale manual.* San Antonio, TX: Psychological Corporation.

Beck, A. T., & Steer, R. A. (1991). *Beck Scale for Suicide Ideation manual.* San Antonio, TX: Harcourt Brace.

Beck, A. T., Steer, R. A., & Ranieri, W. F. (1988). Scale for Suicide Ideation: Psychometric properties of a self-report version. *Journal of Clinical Psychology, 44*(4), 499–505.

Beck, A. T., Weissman, A., Lester, D., & Trexler, L. (1974). The measurement of pessimism: The hopelessness scale. *Journal of Consulting and Clinical Psychology, 42*(6), 861–865.

Belik, S., Cox, B. J., Stein, M. B., Asmundson, G. J. G., & Sareen, J. (2007). Traumatic events and suicidal behavior: Results from a national mental health survey. *Journal of Nervous and Mental Disease, 195*(4), 342–349.

Bender, W. N., Rosenkrans, C. B., & Crane, M. (1999). Stress, depression, and suicide among students with learning disabilities: Assessing the risk. *Learning Disability Quarterly, 22*(2), 143–156.

Berman, A. L. (2006). Risk management with suicidal patients. *Journal of Clinical Psychology, 62*(2), 171–184.

Berman, A. L. (2009). School-based prevention: Research advances and practice implications. *School Psychology Review, 38*(2), 233–238.

Berman, A. L., Jobes, D. A., & Silverman, M. M. (2006). *Adolescent suicide: Assessment and intervention* (2nd ed.). Washington DC: American Psychological Association.

Bierman, K. L., & McCauley, E. (1987). Children's descriptions of their peer interactions: Useful information for clinical child assessment. *Journal of Clinical Child Psychology, 16*(1), 9–18.

Bongar, B., Berman, A. L., Maris, R. W., Silverman, M. M., Harris, E. A., & Packman, W. L. (1998). *Risk management with suicidal patients.* New York: Guilford Press.

Boonstra, H., & Nash, E. (2000). Minors and the right to consent to health care. *The Guttmacher Report on Public Policy, 3*(4), 4–8.

Borowsky, I. W., Resnick, M. D., Ireland, M., & Blum, R. W. (1999). Suicide attempts among American Indian and Alaska Native youth: Risk and protective factors. *Archives of Pediatric Adolescent Medicine, 153*(6), 573–580.

Brausch, A. M., & Gutierrez, P. M. (2010). Differences in non-suicidal self-injury and suicide attempts in adolescents. *Journal of Youth and Adolescence, 39*(3), 233–242.

Brent, D. A., Baugher, M., Bridge, J., Chen, T., & Chiappetta, L. (1999). Age- and sex-related risk factors for adolescent suicide. *Journal of the American Academy of Child and Adolescent Psychiatry, 38*(12), 1497–1505.

Brent, D. A., Johnson, B., Bartle, S., Bridge, J., Rather, C., Matta, J., et al. (1993). Personality disorder, tendency to impulsive violence, and suicidal behavior in adolescents. *Journal of the American Academy of Child and Adolescent Psychiatry, 32*(1), 69–75.

Brent, D. A., Johnson, B. A., Perper, J., Connolly, J., Bridge, J., Bartle, S., et al. (1994). Personality disorder, personality traits, impulsive violence, and completed suicide in adolescents. *Journal of the American Academy of Child and Adolescent Psychiatry, 33*(8), 1080–1086.

Brent, D. A., Kalas, R., Edelbrock, C., & Costello, A. J. (1986). Psychopathology and its relationship to suicidal ideation in childhood and adolescence. *Journal of the American Academy of Child Psychiatry, 25*(5), 666–673.

Brent, D. A., Kerr, M. M., Goldstein, C., & Bozigar, J. (1989). An outbreak of suicide and suicidal behavior in a high school. *Journal of the American Academy of Child and Adolescent Psychiatry, 28*(6), 918–924.

Brent, D. A., Kolko, D. J., Birmaher, B., Baugher, M., Bridge, J., Roth, C., et al. (1998). Predictors of treatment efficacy in a clinical trial of three psychosocial treatments for adolescent depression. *Journal of the American Academy of Child and Adolescent Psychiatry, 37*(9), 906–914.

Brent, D. A., Kolko, D. J., Wartella, M. E., & Boylan, M. B. (1993). Adolescent psychiatric inpatients' risk of suicide attempt at 6-month follow-up. *Journal of the American Academy of Child and Adolescent Psychiatry, 32*(1), 95–105.

Brent, D. A., Perper, J. A., Goldstein, C. E., Kolko, D. J., Allan, M. J., Allman, C. J., et al. (1988). Risk factors for adolescent suicide. A comparison of adolescent suicide victims with suicidal inpatients. *Archives of General Psychiatry, 45*(6), 581–588.

Brent, D. A., Perper, J. A., Moritz, G., Allman, C., Friend, A., Roth, C., et al. (1993). Psychiatric risk factors for adolescent suicide: A case–control study. *Journal of the American Academy of Child and Adolescent Psychiatry, 32*(3), 521–529.

Brent, D. A., Perper, J. A., Moritz, G., & Baugher, M. (1993a). Stressful life events, psychopathology, and adolescent suicide: A case–control study. *Suicide and Life-Threatening Behavior, 23*(3), 179–187.

Brent, D. A., Perper, J. A., Moritz, G., & Baugher, M. (1993b). Suicide in adolescents with no apparent psychopathology. *Journal of the American Academy of Child and Adolescent Psychiatry, 32*(3), 494–500.

Brent, D. A., Perper, J. A., Moritz, G., & Liotus, L. (1994). Familial risk factors for adolescent suicide: A case–control study. *Acta Psychiatrica Scandinavica, 89*(1), 52–58.

Britto, M. T., Klostermann, B. K., Bonny, A. E., Altum, S. A., & Hornung, R. W. (2001). Impact of a school-based intervention on access to healthcare for underserved youth. *Journal of Adolescent Health, 29*(2), 116–124.

Brown, G. K., Ten Have, T. R., Henriques, G. R., Xie, S. X., Hollander, J. E., & Beck, A. T. (2005). Cognitive therapy for the prevention of suicide attempts: A randomized controlled trial. *Journal of the American Medical Association, 294*(5), 563–570.

Brown, R. T., Antonuccio, D. O., DuPaul, G. J., Fristad, M. A., King, C. A., Leslie, L. K., et al. (2008). *Childhood mental health disorders: Evidence base and contextual factors for psychological, psychopharmacological, and combined interventions.* Washington, DC: American Psychological Association.

Bryan, C. J., & Rudd, M. D. (2006). Advances in the assessment of suicide risk. *Journal of Clinical Psychology, 62*(2), 185–200.

Centers for Disease Control and Prevention. (2011). *2011 State and Local Youth Risk Behavior Survey.* Retrieved December 19, 2012, from www.cdc.gov/healthyyouth/yrbs/pdf/questionnaire/2009HighSchool.pdf

Centers for Disease Control and Prevention. (2012a). *Web-based Injury Statistics Query and Reporting System (WISQARS).* Retrieved May 11, 2012, from *www.cdc.gov/ncipc/wisqars.*

Centers for Disease Control and Prevention. (2012b). *Youth Risk Behavior Surveillance—United States, 2011.* Retrieved October 22, 2012, from *www.cdc.gov/mmwr/pdf/ss/ss6104.pdf.*

Chemtob, C. M., Hamada, R. S., Bauer, G., Kinney, B., & Torigoe, R.

Y. (1988). Patients' suicides: Frequency and impact on psychiatrists. *American Journal of Psychiatry, 145*(2), 224–228.

Chemtob, C. M., Hamada, R. S., Bauer, G., Torigoe, R. Y., & Kinney, B. (1988). Patient suicide: Frequency and impact on psychologists. *Professional Psychology: Research and Practice, 19*(4), 416–420.

Claassen, C. A., & Larkin, G. L. (2005). Occult suicidality in an emergency department population. *The British Journal of Psychiatry, 186*(4), 352–353.

Conwell, Y., Duberstein, P. R., Cox, C., Herrmann, J. H., Forbes, N. T., & Caine, E. D. (1996). Relationships of age and axis I diagnoses in victims of completed suicide: A psychological autopsy study. *American Journal of Psychiatry, 153*(8), 1001–1008.

Corcoran, J., Dattalo, P., Crowley, M., Brown, E., & Grindle, L. (2011). A systematic review of psychosocial interventions for suicidal adolescents. *Children and Youth Services Review, 33*(11), 2112–2118.

Costello, E. J., Angold, A., Cicchetti, D., & Cohen, D. J. (2006). Developmental epidemiology. In D. Cicchetti & D. J. Cohen (Eds.), *Developmental psychopathology, Vol 1: Theory and method* (2nd ed., pp. 41–75). Hoboken, NJ: Wiley.

Cronholm, P. F., Barg, F. K., Pailler, M. E., Wintersteen, M. B., Diamond, G. S., & Fein, J. A. (2010). Adolescent depression: Views of health care providers in a pediatric emergency department. *Pediatric Emergency Care, 26*(2), 111.

Crosby, A. E., Ortega, L., & Melanson, C. (2011). *Self-directed violence surveillance: Uniform definitions and recommended data elements, Version 1.0.* Atlanta: Centers for Disease Control and Prevention, National Center for Injury Prevention and Control.

Cuffe, S. P., Waller, J. L., Addy, C. L., McKeown, R. E., Jackson, K. L., Moloo, J., et al. (2001). A longitudinal study of adolescent mental health service use. *The Journal of Behavioral Health Services and Research, 28*(1), 1–11.

Cumsille, P. E., & Epstein, N. (1994). Family cohesion, family adaptability, social support, and adolescent depressive symptoms in outpatient clinic families. *Journal of Family Psychology, 8*(2), 202–214.

D'Augelli, A. R., Grossman, A. H., Salter, N. P., Vasey, J. J., Starks, M. T., & Sinclair, K. O. (2005). Predicting the suicide attempts of lesbian, gay, and bisexual youth. *Suicide and Life-Threatening Behavior, 35*(6), 646–660.

D'Augelli, A. R., Hershberger, S. L., & Pilkington, N. W. (2001). Suicidality patterns and sexual orientation-related factors among lesbian, gay, and bisexual youths. *Suicide and Life-Threatening Behavior, 31*(3), 250–264.

Daniel, S. S., & Goldston, D. B. (2009). Interventions for suicidal youth: A review of the literature and developmental considerations. *Suicide and Life-Threatening Behavior, 39*(3), 252–268.

Daniel, S. S., Walsh, A. K., Goldston, D. B., Arnold, E. M., Reboussin, B. A., & Wood, F. B. (2006). Suicidality, school dropout, and reading problems among adolescents. *Journal of Learning Disabilities, 39*(6), 507–514.

Davies, M., & Cunningham, G. (1999). Adolescent parasuicide in the Foyle area. *Irish Journal of Psychological Medicine, 16*(1), 9-12.

David-Ferdon, C., & Kaslow, N. J. (2008). Evidence-based psychosocial treatments for child and adolescent depression. *Journal of Clinical Child and Adolescent Psychology, 37*(1), 62–104.

DeJong, T. M., & Overholser, J. C. (2009). Assessment of depression and suicidal actions: Agreement between suicide attempters and informant reports. *Suicide and Life-Threatening Behavior, 39*(1), 38–46.

Delfabbro, P., Winefield, T., Trainor, S., Dollard, M., Anderson, S., Metzer, J., et al. (2006). Peer and teacher bullying/victimization of South Australian secondary school students: Prevalence and psychosocial profiles. *British Journal of Educational Psychology, 76*(1), 71–90.

Diamond, G., Levy, S., Bevans, K. B., Fein, J. A., Wintersteen, M. B., Tien, A., et al. (2010). Development, validation, and utility of internet-based, behavioral health screen for adolescents. *Pediatrics, 126*(1), e163–e170.

Dubow, E. F., Kausch, D. F., Blum, M. C., Reed, J., & Bush, E. (1989). Correlates of suicidal ideation and attempts in a community sample of junior high and high school students. *Journal of Clinical Child Psychology, 18*(2), 158–166.

East, P. L., Hess, L. E., & Lerner, R. M. (1987). Peer social support and adjustment of early adolescent peer groups. *Journal of Early Adolescence, 7*(2), 153–163.

Eckert, T. L., Miller, D. N., DuPaul, G. J., & Riley-Tillman, T. C. (2003). Adolescent suicide prevention: School psychologists' acceptability of school-based programs. *School Psychology Review, 32*(1), 57–76.

Eckert, T. L., Miller, D. N., Riley-Tillman, T. C., & DuPaul, G. J. (2006). Adolescent suicide prevention: Gender differences in students' perceptions of the acceptability and intrusiveness of school-based screening programs. *Journal of School Psychology, 44*(4), 271–285.

Esposito-Smythers, C., & Spirito, A. (2004). Adolescent substance use and suicidal behavior: A review with implications for treatment research. *Alcoholism: Clinical and Experimental Research, 28,* 77S–88S.

Esposito-Smythers, C., Spirito, A., Kahler, C. W., Hunt, J., & Monti, P. (2011). Treatment of co-occurring substance abuse and suicidality among adolescents: A randomized trial. *Journal of Consulting and Clinical Psychology, 79*(6):728–739.

Fein, J. A., Pailler, E. P., Barg, F. K., Wintersteen, M. B. H., K., Tien, A., & Diamond, G. S. (2010). Feasibility and effects of a web-based adolescent psychiatric assessment administered by clinical staff in the pediatric emergency department. *Archives of Pediatric and Adolescent Medicine, 164*(12), 1112–1117.

Fergusson, D. M., Woodward, L. J., & Horwood, L. J. (2000). Risk factors and life processes associated with the onset of suicidal behaviour during adolescence and early adulthood. *Psychological Medicine, 30*(1), 23–39.

Folse, V. N., Eich, K. N., Hall, A. M., & Ruppman, J. B. (2006). Detecting suicide risk in adolescents and adults in an emergency department: A pilot study. *Journal of Psychosocial Nursing and Mental Health Services, 44*(3), 22–29.

Fotheringham, M. J., & Sawyer, M. G. (1995). Do adolescents know where to find help for mental health problems? A brief report. *Journal of Paediatrics and Child Health, 31*(1), 41–43.

Frankenfield, D. L., Keyl, P. M., Gielen, A., Wissow, L. S., Werthamer, L., & Baker, S. P. (2000). Adolescent patients—healthy or hurting?: Missed opportunities to screen for suicide risk in the primary care setting. *Archives of Pediatrics and Adolescent Medicine, 154*(2), 162–168.

Fristad, M. A., Verducci, J. S., Walters, K., & Young, M. E. (2009). Impact of multifamily psychoeducational psychotherapy in treating children aged 8 to 12 years with mood disorders. *Archives of General Psychiatry, 66*(9), 1013–1020.

Garlow, S. J., Rosenberg, J., Moore, J. D., Haas, A. P., Koestner, B., Hendin, H., et al. (2008). Depression, desperation, and suicidal ideation in college students: Results from the American Foundation for Suicide Prevention College Screening Project at Emory University. *Depression and Anxiety, 25*(6), 482–488.

Garofalo, R., Wolf, R. C., Wissow, L. S., Woods, E. R., & Goodman, E. (1999). Sexual orientation and risk of suicide attempts among a representative sample of youth. *Archives of Pediatrics and Adolescent Medicine, 153*(5), 487–493.

Giaconia, R. M., Reinherz, H. Z., Silverman, A. B., & Pakiz, B. (1995). Traumas and posttraumatic stress disorder in a community population of older adolescents. *Journal of the American Academy of Child and Adolescent Psychiatry, 34*(10), 1369–1380.

Goldstein, M. J. (1978). Drug and family therapy in the aftercare of acute schizophrenics. *Archives of General Psychiatry, 35*(10), 1169–1177.

Goldstein, T. R., Birmaher, B., Axelson, D., Ryan, N. D., Strober, M. A., Gill, M. K., et al. (2005). History of suicide attempts in pediatric bipolar disorder: Factors associated with increased risk. *Bipolar Disorders, 7*(6), 525–535.

Goldstein, T. R., Bridge, J. A., & Brent, D. A. (2008). Sleep disturbance preceding completed suicide in adolescents. *Journal of Consulting and Clinical Psychology, 76*(1), 84–91.

Goldston, D. B. (2003). *Measuring suicidal behavior and risk in children and adolescents.* Washington, DC: American Psychological Association.

Goldston, D. B., Daniel, S. S., Reboussin, B. A., Reboussin, D. M., Frazier, P. H., & Harris, A. E. (2001). Cognitive risk factors and suicide attempts among formerly hospitalized adolescents: A prospective naturalistic study. *Journal of the American Academy of Child and Adolescent Psychiatry, 40*(1), 91–99.

Goldston, D. B., Daniel, S. S., Reboussin, D. M., Reboussin, B. A., Frazier, P. H., & Kelley, A. E. (1999). Suicide attempts among formerly hospitalized adolescents: A prospective naturalistic study of risk during the first 5 years after discharge. *Journal of the American Academy of Child and Adolescent Psychiatry, 38*(6), 660–671.

Goldston, D. B., Daniel, S. S., Reboussin, D. M., Reboussin, B. A., Kelley, A. E., & Frazier, P. H. (1998). Psychiatric diagnoses of previous suicide attempters, first-time attempters, and repeat attempters on an adolescent inpatient psychiatry unit. *Journal of the American Academy of Child and Adolescent Psychiatry, 37*(9), 924–932.

Gould, M. S., Fisher, P., Parides, M., Flory, M., & Shaffer, D. (1996). Psychosocial risk factors of child and adolescent completed suicide. *Archives of General Psychiatry, 53*(12), 1155–1162.

Gould, M. S., Greenberg, T., Velting, D. M., & Shaffer, D. (2003). Youth suicide risk and preventive interventions: A review of the past 10 years. *Journal of the American Academy of Child and Adolescent Psychiatry, 42*(4), 386–405.

Gould, M. S., Hendin, H., & Mann, J. J. (2001). Suicide and the media. In H. Hendin & J. J. Mann (Eds.), *The clinical science of suicide prevention* (pp. 200–224). New York: New York Academy of Sciences.

Gould, M. S., King, R. A., Greenwald, S., Fisher, P., Schwab-Stone, M., Kramer, R., et al. (1998). Psychopathology associated with suicidal ideation and attempts among children and adolescents. *Journal of the American Academy of Child and Adolescent Psychiatry, 37*(9), 915–923.

Gould, M. S., Marrocco, F. A., Hoagwood, K., Kleinman, M., Amakawa, L., & Altschuler, E. (2009). Service use by at-risk youths after school-based suicide screening. *Journal of the American Academy of Child and Adolescent Psychiatry, 48*(12), 1193–1201.

Gould, M. S., Marrocco, F. A., Kleinman, M., Thomas, J. G., Mostkoff, K., Cote, J., et al. (2005). Evaluating iatrogenic risk of youth suicide screening programs: A randomized controlled trial. *Journal of the American Medical Association, 293*(13), 1635–1643.

Gould, M. S., Wallenstein, S., & Kleinman, M. (1990). Time–space clustering of teenage suicide. *American Journal of Epidemiology, 131*(1), 71–78.

Grossman, D. C., Milligan, B. C., & Deyo, R. A. (1991). Risk factors for suicide attempts among Navajo adolescents. *American Journal of Public Health, 81*(7), 870–874.

Groves, S. A., Stanley, B. H., & Sher, L. (2007). Ethnicity and the relationship between adolescent alcohol use and suicidal behavior. *International Journal of Adolescent Medicine and Health, 19*(1), 19–25.

Gutheil, T. G. (1980). Paranoia and progress notes: A guide to forensically informed psychiatric recordkeeping. *Hospital and Community Psychiatry, 31*(7), 479–482.

Hallfors, D. D., Waller, M. W., Ford, C. A., Halpern, C. T., Brodish, P. H., & Iritani, B. (2004). Adolescent depression and suicide risk: Association with sex and drug behavior. *American Journal of Preventive Medicine, 27*(3), 224–230.

Hamann, C. J., Larkin, G. L., Brown, B., Schwann, C., & George, V. (2007). Differences in computer prompted self-report and physician-elicited responses in screening of emergency department patients for substance use and abuse. *Annals of Emergency Medicine, 50*(3, Suppl. 1), S43–S43.

Haynie, D. L., South, S. J., & Bose, S. (2006). Residential mobility and attempted suicide among adolescents: An individual-level analysis. *Sociological Quarterly, 47*(4), 693–721.

Heath, A. C., Howells, W., Bucholz, K. K., Glowinski, A. L., Nelson, E. C., & Madden, P. A. F. (2002). Ascertainment of a midwestern U.S. female adolescent twin cohort for alcohol studies: Assessment of sample representativeness using birth record data. *Twin Research, 5*(2), 107–112.

Heila, H., Isometsa, E. T., Henriksson, M. M., Heikkinen, M. E., Marttunen, M. J., & Lonnqvist, J. K. (1997). Suicide and schizophrenia: A nationwide psychological autopsy study on age- and sex-specific clinical characteristics of 92 suicide victims with schizophrenia. *American Journal of Psychiatry, 154*(9), 1235–1242.

Horesh, N., Gothelf, D., Ofek, H., Weizman, T., & Apter, A. (1999). Impulsivity as a correlate of suicidal behavior in adolescent psychiatric inpatients. *Crisis: The Journal of Crisis Intervention and Suicide Prevention, 20*(1), 8–14.

Horowitz, L. M., Ballard, E., Teach, S., J., Bosk, A., Robensteing, D., L., Paramjit, J., et al. (2010). Feasibility of screening patients with nonpsychiatric complaints for suicide risk in pediatric emergency department. *Pediatric Emergency Care, 26*(11), 787–792.

Horowitz, L. M., Wang, P. S., Koocher, G. P., Burr, B. H., Smith, M. F., Klavon, S., & Cleary, P. D. (2001). Detecting suicide risk in a pediatric emergency department: Development of a brief screening tool. *Pediatrics, 107*(5), 1133-1137.

Husky, M. M., McGuire, L., Flynn, L., Chrostowski, C., & Olfson, M. (2009). Correlates of help-seeking behavior among at-risk adolescents. *Child Psychiatry and Human Development, 40*(1), 15–24.

Huth-Bocks, A. C., Kerr, D. C. R., Ivey, A. Z., Kramer, A. C., & King, C. A. (2007). Assessment of psychiatrically hospitalized suicidal adolescents: Self-report instruments as predictors of suicidal thoughts and behavior. *Journal of the American Academy of Child and Adolescent Psychiatry, 46*(3), 387–395.

Jacob, S. (2009). Putting it all together: Implications for school psychology. *School Psychology Review, 38*(2), 239–243.

Jessor, R. (1991). Risk behavior in adolescence: A psychosocial framework for understanding and action. *Journal of Adolescent Health, 12*(8), 597–605.

Jobes, D. A. (2006). *Managing suicidal risk: A collaborative approach.* New York: Guilford Press.

Jobes, D. A., & Maltsberger, J. T. (1995). The hazards of treating suicidal patients. In M. B. Sussman (Ed.), *A perilous calling: The hazards of psychotherapy practice* (pp. 200–214). Oxford UK: Wiley.

Johnson, J. G., Cohen, P., Gould, M. S., Kasen, S., Brown, J., & Brook, J. S. (2002). Childhood adversities, interpersonal difficulties, and risk for suicide attempts during late adolescence and early adulthood. *Archives of General Psychiatry, 59*(8), 741–749.

Kalafat, J. (2003). School approaches to youth suicide prevention. *American Behavioral Scientist, 46*(9), 1211–1223.

Kalafat, J., & Elias, M. (1992). Adolescents' experience with and response to suicidal peers. *Suicide and Life-Threatening Behavior, 22*, 315–321.

Kaltiala-Heino, R., Rimpelä, M., Marttunen, M. J., Rimpelä, A., & Rantanen, P. (1999). Bullying, depression, and suicidal ideation in Finnish adolescents: School survey. *British Medical Journal, 319*(7206), 348–351.

Karver, M. S., Handelsman, J. B., Fields, S., & Bickman, L. (2006). Meta-analysis of therapeutic relationship variables in youth and family therapy: The evidence for different relationship variables in the child and adolescent treatment outcome literature. *Clinical Psychology Review, 26*(1), 50–65.

Kashden, J., Fremouw, W. J., Callahan, T. S., & Franzen, M. D. (1993). Impulsivity in suicidal and nonsuicidal adolescents. *Journal of Abnormal Child Psychology, 21*(3), 339–353.

Kaufman, J., Birmaher, B., Brent, D. A., & Rao, U. (1997). Schedule for Affective Disorders and Schizophrenia for School-Age Children—Present and Lifetime version (K-SADS-PL): Initial reliability and validity data. *Journal of the American Academy of Child and Adolescent Psychiatry, 36*(7), 980–988.

Kautz, C., Mauch, D., & Smith, S. A. (2008). *Reimbursement of mental health services in primary care settings* (HHS Pub. No. SMA-08-4324). Rockville, MD: Center for Mental Health Services, Substance Abuse and Mental Health Services Administration.

Kerr, D. C. R., Preuss, L. J., & King, C. A. (2006). Suicidal adolescents' social support from family and peers: Gender-specific associations with psychopathology. *Journal of Abnormal Child Psychology, 34*(1), 103–114.

Kim, Y. S., & Leventhal, B. (2008). Bullying and suicide: A review. *International Journal of Adolescent Medicine and Health, 20*(2), 133–154.

King, C. A. (1997). Suicidal behavior in adolescence. In R. Maris, M. Silverman, & S. Canetto (Eds.), *Review of suicidology, 1997* (pp. 61–95). New York: Guilford Press.

King, C. A., Gipson, P. Y., Agarwala, P., & Opperman, K. J. (November

2011). *Using the C-SSRS to assess adolescents in psychiatric emergency settings: Predictive validity across a one-year period.* Paper presented at the National Network of Depression Centers Annual Conference, Baltimore, MD.

King, C. A., Hovey, J. D., Brand, E., & Ghaziuddin, N. (1997). Prediction of positive outcomes for adolescent psychiatric inpatients. *Journal of the American Academy of Child and Adolescent Psychiatry, 36*(10), 1434–1442.

King, C. A., Hovey, J. D., Brand, E., & Wilson, R. (1997). Suicidal adolescents after hospitalization: Parent and family impacts on treatment follow-through. *Journal of the American Academy of Child and Adolescent Psychiatry, 36*(1), 85–93.

King, C. A., Jiang, Q., Czyz, E., & Kerr, D. C. R. (2012). *Twelve-month predictive validity of suicidal ideation for psychiatrically hospitalized adolescent boys and girls.* Manuscript submitted for publication.

King, C. A., Klaus, N. M., Kramer, A., Venkataraman, S., Quinlan, P., & Gillespie, B. (2009). The Youth Nominated Support Team for suicidal adolescents—version II: A randomized control intervention trial. *Journal of Consulting and Clinical Psychology, 77*(5), 880–893.

King, C. A., & Merchant, C. R. (2008). Social and interpersonal factors relating to adolescent suicidality: A review of the literature. *Archives of Suicide Research, 12*(3), 181–196.

King, C. A., O'Mara, R. M., Hayward, C. N., & Cunningham, R. M. (2009). Adolescent suicide risk screening in the emergency department. *Academic Emergency Medicine, 16*(11), 1234–1241.

King, C. A., Segal, H. G., Kaminski, K., & Naylor, M. W. (1995). A prospective study of adolescent suicidal behavior following hospitalization. *Suicide and Life-Threatening Behavior, 25*(3), 327–338.

King, C. A., Segal, H. G., Naylor, M. W., & Evans, T. (1993). Family functioning and suicidal behavior in adolescent inpatients with mood disorders. *Journal of the American Academy of Child and Adolescent Psychiatry, 32*(6), 1198–1206.

Klaus, N. M., & Fristad, M. A. (2005). Family psychoeducation as a valuable adjunctive intervention for children with bipolar disorder. *Directions in Psychiatry, 25*(3), 217–230.

Klaus, N. M., Mobilio, A., & King, C. A. (2009). Parent–adolescent agreement concerning adolescents' suicidal thoughts and behaviors. *Journal of Clinical Child and Adolescent Psychology, 38*(2), 245–255.

Kleespies, P. M., Penk, W. E., & Forsyth, J. P. (1993). The stress of patient suicidal behavior during clinical training: Incidence, impact, and recovery. *Professional Psychology: Research and Practice, 24*(3), 293–303.

Klimes-Dougan, B. (1998). Screening for suicidal ideation in children and adolescents: Methodological considerations. *Journal of Adolescence, 21*(4), 435–444.

Klomek, A. B., Marrocco, F., Kleinman, M., Schonfeld, I. S., & Gould, M. (2007). Bullying, depression, and suicidality in adolescents. *Journal of the American Academy of Child and Adolescent Psychiatry, 46,* 40–49.

Klonsky, E. D. (2007). The functions of deliberate self-injury: A review of the evidence. *Clinical Psychology Review, 27*(2), 226–239.

Kruesi, M. J. P., Grossman, J., Pennington, J. M., Woodward, P. J., Duda, D., & Hirsch, J. G. (1999). Suicide and violence prevention: Parent education in the emergency department. *Journal of the American Academy of Child and Adolescent Psychiatry, 38*(3), 250–255.

La Greca, A. M., & Lopez, N. (1998). Social anxiety among adolescents: Linkages with peer relations and friendships. *Journal of Abnormal Child Psychology, 26*(2), 83–94.

LaFromboise, T., & Howard-Pitney, B. (1995). The Zuni life skills development curriculum: Description and evaluation of a suicide prevention program. *Journal of Counseling Psychology, 42*(4), 479–486.

Lewinsohn, P. M., Rohde, P., & Seeley, J. R. (1994). Psychosocial risk factors for future adolescent suicide attempts. *Journal of Consulting and Clinical Psychology, 62*(2), 297–305.

Lewinsohn, P. M., Rohde, P., & Seeley, J. R. (1996). Adolescent suicidal ideation and attempts: Prevalence, risk factors, and clinical implications. *Clinical Psychology: Science and Practice, 3*(1), 25–46.

Lewinsohn, P. M., Rohde, P., Seeley, J. R., & Baldwin, C. L. (2001). Gender differences in suicide attempts from adolescence to young adulthood. *Journal of the American Academy of Child and Adolescent Psychiatry, 40*(4), 427–434.

Li, X., & Phillips, M. R. (2008). Using in-depth interviewing methods with suicide attempters and their associates to assess their ideas about the characteristics and causes of the attempt. *Chinese Mental Health Journal, 22*(1), 43–50.

Liang, H., Flisher, A. J., & Lombard, C. J. (2007). Bullying, violence, and risk behavior in South African school students. *Child Abuse and Neglect, 31*(2), 161–171.

Linehan, M. M. (2011). Dialectical behavior therapy and telephone coaching. *Cognitive and Behavioral Practice, 18*(2), 207–208.

Linehan, M. M., Comtois, K. A., Murray, A. M., Brown, M. Z., Gallop, R. J., Heard, H. L., et al. (2006). Two-year randomized controlled trial and follow-up of dialectical behavior therapy vs. therapy by experts for suicidal behaviors and borderline personality disorder. *Archives of General Psychiatry, 63*(7), 757–766.

Liu, R. T., & Mustanski, B. (2012). Suicidal ideation and self-harm in lesbian, gay, bisexual, and transgender youth. *American Journal of Preventive Medicine, 42*(3), 221-228.

Liu, X. (2004). Sleep and Adolescent Suicidal Behavior. *Sleep: Journal of Sleep and Sleep Disorders Research, 27*(7), 1351–1358.

Lowenstein, S. R., Koziol-McLain, J., Thompson, M., Bernstein, E., Greenberg, K., Gerson, L. W., et al. (1998). Behavioral risk factors in emergency department patients: A multisite survey. *Academic Emergency Medicine, 5*(8), 781–787.

Luoma, J. B., Martin, C. E., & Pearson, J. L. (2002). Contact with mental health and primary care providers before suicide: A review of the evidence. *American Journal of Psychiatry, 159*(6), 909–916.

Mahon, N. E., Yarcheski, A., Yarcheski, T. J., Cannella, B. L., & Hanks, M. M. (2006). A meta-analytic study of predictors for loneliness during adolescence. *Nursing Research, 55*(5), 308–315.

Mann, J. J., Apter, A., Bertolote, J., Beautrais, A. L., Currier, D., Haas, A., et al. (2005). Suicide prevention strategies: A systematic review. *Journal of the American Medical Association, 294*(16), 2064–2074.

Marcell, A. V., & Halpern-Felsher, B. L. (2005). Adolescents' health beliefs are critical in their intentions to seek physician care. *Preventive Medicine, 41*(1), 118–125.

Martin, A. & Volkmar, F. R. (2007). *Lewis's Child and Adolescent Psychiatry*. Philadelphia, PA: Lippincott Williams & Wilkins.

Martin, G., Bergen, H. A., Richardson, A. S., Roeger, L., & Allison, S. (2004). Sexual abuse and suicidality: Gender differences in a large community sample of adolescents. *Child Abuse and Neglect, 28*(5), 491–503.

Marttunen, M. J., Aro, H. M., Henriksson, M. M., & Lonnqvist, J. K. (1991). Mental disorders in adolescent suicide: DSM-III–R Axes I and II diagnoses in suicides among 13 to 19-year-olds in Finland. *Archives of General Psychiatry, 48*(9), 834–839.

Marttunen, M. J., Aro, H. M., & Lonnqvist, J. K. (1992). Adolescent suicide: Endpoint of long-term difficulties. *Journal of the American Academy of Child and Adolescent Psychiatry, 31*(4), 649–654.

Mazza, J. J., & Reynolds, W. M. (1998). A longitudinal investigation of depression, hopelessness, social support, and major and minor life events and their relation to suicidal ideation in adolescents. *Suicide and Life-Threatening Behavior, 28*(4), 358–374.

McGuffin, P., Marusic, A., & Farmer, A. (2001). What can psychiatric genetics offer suicidology? *Crisis: The Journal of Crisis Intervention and Suicide Prevention, 22*(2), 61–65.

McKeown, R. E., Garrison, C. Z., Cuffe, S. P., Waller, J. L., Jackson, K. L., & Addy, C. L. (1998). Incidence and predictors of suicidal behaviors in a longitudinal sample of young adolescents. *Journal of the American Academy of Child and Adolescent Psychiatry, 37*(6), 612–619.

McKnight-Eily, L. R., Eaton, D. K., Lowry, R., Croft, J. B., Presley-Cantrell, L., & Perry, G. S. (2011). Relationships between hours of sleep and health-risk behaviors in US adolescent students. *Preventive Medicine, 53*(4–5), 271–273.

McManus, B. L., Kruesi, M. J., Dontes, A. E., Defazio, C. R., Piotrowski, J. T., & Woodward, P. J. (1997). Child and adolescent suicide attempts: An opportunity for emergency departments to provide injury prevention education. *American Journal of Emergency Medicine, 15*(4), 357–360.

Meehan, J., Kapur, N., Hunt, I. M., Turnbull, P., Robinson, J., Bickley, H., et al. (2006). Suicide in mental health inpatients and within 3 months of discharge: National clinical survey. *British Journal of Psychiatry, 188*(2), 129–134.

Melanie Bellah et al. v. Daniel P. Greenson. , 81 Cal. App. 3d 614 (1978).

Mendenhall, A. N., Fristad, M. A., & Early, T. J. (2009). Factors influencing service utilization and mood symptom severity in children with mood disorders: Effects of multifamily psychoeducation groups (MFPGs). *Journal of Consulting and Clinical Psychology, 77*(3), 463–473.

Merikangas, K. R., He, J., Burstein, M., Swendsen, J., Avenevoli, S., Case, B., et al. (2011). Service utilization for lifetime mental disorders in U.S. adolescents: Results of the National Comorbidity Survey–Adolescent Supplement (NCSA). *Journal of the American Academy of Child and Adolescent Psychiatry, 50*(1), 32–45.

Miklowitz, D. J., Simoneau, T. L., George, E. L., Richards, J. A., Kalbag, A., Sachs-Ericsson, N., et al. (2000). Family-focused treatment of bipolar disorder: 1-year effects of a psychoeducational program in conjunction with pharmacotherapy. *Biological Psychiatry, 48*(6), 582–592.

Miller, A. L., Rathus, J. H., & Linehan, M. M. (2007). *Dialectical behavior therapy with suicidal adolescents*. New York: Guilford Press.

Miller, D. N., & Jome, L. M. (2008). School psychologists and the assessment of childhood internalizing disorders: Perceived knowledge, role preferences and training needs. *School Psychology International, 29*(4), 500–510.

Moscicki, E. K. (1995). Epidemiology of suicidal behavior. *Suicide and Life-Threatening Behavior, 25*(1), 22–35.

MTA Cooperative Group. (1999). Moderators and mediators of treatment response for children with attention-deficit/hyperactivity disorder. *Archives of General Psychiatry, 56*, 1088–1096.

Muehlenkamp, J. J., & Gutierrez, P. M. (2004). An investigation of differences between self-injurious behavior and suicide attempts in a sample of adolescents. *Suicide and Life-Threatening Behavior, 34*(1), 12–23.

Muehlenkamp, J. J., & Gutierrez, P. M. (2007). Risk for suicide attempts among adolescents who engage in non-suicidal self-injury. *Archives of Suicide Research, 11*(1), 69–82.

Myers, K., McCauley, E., Calderon, R., & Treder, R. (1991). The 3-year longitudinal course of suicidality and predictive factors for subsequent suicidality in youths with major depressive disorder. *Journal of the American Academy of Child and Adolescent Psychiatry, 30*(5), 804–810.

National Association of Social Workers. (2009). *Making the case for evidence-based practice*. Retrieved May 16, 2012, from *www.socialworkers.org/practice/adolescent_health/shift/case.asp*.

National Institute for Clinical Excellence, National Collaborating Centre for Mental Health. (2004). *Self-harm: The short-term physical and psychological management and secondary prevention of self-harm in primary and secondary care*. Retrieved from *www.nice.org.uk/nicemedia/live/10946/29424/29424.pdf*

National Research Council and Institute of Medicine of the National Academies. (2009). *Preventing mental, emotional, and behavioral disorders among young people: Progress and possibilities*. Washington, DC: The National Academies Press.

Neumark-Sztainer, D., Story, M., Dixon, L. B., & Murray, D. M. (1998). Adolescents engaging in unhealthy weight-control behaviors: Are they at risk for other health-compromising behaviors? *American Journal of Public Health, 88*(6), 952–955.

New Freedom Commission on Mental Health. (2003). Achieving a promise: Transforming mental health care in America: *Executive summary* (Pub No. SMA-03-3831). Rockville, MD: Department of Health and Human Services.

Nock, M. K., Joiner, T. E., Jr., Gordon, K. H., Lloyd-Richardson, E., & Prinstein, M. J. (2006). Non-suicidal self-injury among adolescents: Diagnostic correlates and relation to suicide attempts. *Psychiatry Research, 144*(1), 65–72.

O'Carroll, P. W., Berman, A., Maris, R. W., & Moscicki, E. K. (1996). Beyond the tower of Babel: A nomenclature for suicidology. *Suicide and Life-Threatening Behavior, 26*(3), 237–252.

O'Donnell, L., Stueve, A., Wardlaw, D., & O'Donnell, C. (2003). Adolescent suicidality and adult support: The Reach for Health study of urban youth. *American Journal of Health Behavior, 27*(6), 633–644.

O'Mara, R. M., Hill, R. M., Cunningham, R. M., & King, C. A. (2012). Adolescent and parent attitudes toward screening for suicide risk and mental health problems in the pediatric emergency department. *Pediatric Emergency Care, 28*(7), 626-632.

Olson, A. L., Kemper, K. J., Kelleher, K. J., Hammond, C. S., Zuckerman, B. S., & Dietrich, A. J. (2002). Primary care pediatricians' roles and perceived responsibilities in the identification and management of maternal depression. *Pediatrics, 110*(6), 1169–1176.

Packman, W. L., & Harris, E. A. (1998). Legal issues and risk management in suicidal patients. In B. Bongar, A. L. Berman, R. W. Maris, M. M. Silverman, E. A. Harris, & W. L. Packman (Eds.), *Risk management with suicidal patients* (pp. 150–186). New York: Guilford Press.

Pailler, M. E., Cronholm, P. F., Barg, F. K., Wintersteen, M. B., Diamond, G. S., & Fein, J. A. (2009). Patients' and caregivers' beliefs about depression screening and referral in the emergency department. *Pediatric Emergency Care, 25*(11), 721–727.

Palmer, B. A., Pankratz, V. S., & Bostwick, J. M. (2005). The lifetime risk of suicide in schizophrenia: A reexamination. *Archives of General Psychiatry, 62*(3), 247–253.

Panagioti, M., Gooding, P., & Tarrier, N. (2009). Posttraumatic stress disorder and suicidal behavior: A narrative review. *Clinical Psychology Review, 29*(6), 471–482.

Park, H. S., Schepp, K. G., Jang, E. H., & Koo, H. Y. (2006). Predictors of suicidal ideation among high school students by gender in South Korea. *Journal of School Health, 76*(5), 181–188.

Pealer, L. N., Weiler, R. M., Pigg, R. M., Jr., Miller, D., & Dorman, S. M.

(2001). The feasibility of a web-based surveillance system to collect health risk behavior data from college students. *Health Education and Behavior, 29*(5), 547–559.

Pena, J. B., & Caine, E. D. (2006). Screening as an approach for adolescent suicide prevention. *Suicide and Life-Threatening Behavior, 36*(6), 614–637.

Pena, J. B., Matthieu, M. M., Zayas, L. H., Masyn, K. E., & Caine, E. D. (2012). Co-occurring risk behaviors among white, black, and Hispanic U.S. high school adolescents with suicide attempts requiring medical attention, 1999–2007: Implications for future prevention initiatives. *Social Psychiatry and Psychiatric Epidemiology, 47*(1), 29–42.

Perkins, D. F., & Hartless, G. (2002). An ecological risk-factor examination of suicide ideation and behavior of adolescents. *Journal of Adolescent Research, 17*(1), 3–26.

Peters, R. D. (1988). Mental health promotion in children and adolescents: An emerging role for psychology. *Canadian Journal of Behavioural Science, 20*(4), 389–401.

Pfeffer, C. R., Klerman, G. L., Hurt, S. W., & Kakuma, T. (1993). Suicidal children grow up: Rates and psychosocial risk factors for suicide attempts during follow-up. *Journal of the American Academy of Child and Adolescent Psychiatry, 32*(1), 106–113.

Pfeffer, C. R., Newcorn, J. H., Kaplan, G., & Mizruchi, M. S. (1988). Suicidal behavior in adolescent psychiatric inpatients. *Journal of the American Academy of Child and Adolescent Psychiatry, 27*(3), 357–361.

Pfeffer, C. R., Normandin, L., & Kakuma, T. (1994). Suicidal children grow up: Suicidal behavior and psychiatric disorders among relatives. *Journal of the American Academy of Child and Adolescent Psychiatry, 33*(8), 1087–1097.

Pilowsky, D. J., Wu, L.-T., & Anthony, J. C. (1999). Panic attacks and suicide attempts in mid-adolescence. *American Journal of Psychiatry, 156*(10), 1545–1549.

Pokorny, A. D. (1983). Prediction of suicide in psychiatric patients: Report of a prospective study. *Archives of General Psychiatry, 40*(3), 249–257.

Pompili, M., Mancinelli, I., & Tatarelli, R. (2003). Stigma as a cause of suicide. *British Journal of Psychiatry, 183*(2), 173–174.

Posner, K., Brown, G. K., Stanley, B., Brent, D. A., Yershova, K. V., Oquendo, M. A., et al. (2011). The Columbia–Suicide Severity Rating

Scale: Initial validity and internal consistency findings from three multisite studies with adolescents and adults. *American Journal of Psychiatry, 168*(12), 1266–1277.

Posner, K., Oquendo, M. A., Gould, M., Stanley, B., & Davies, M. (2007). Columbia Classification Algorithm of Suicide Assessment (C-CASA): Classification of suicidal events in the FDA's pediatric suicidal risk analysis of antidepressants. *American Journal of Psychiatry, 164*(7), 1035–1043.

Prinstein, M. J., Boergers, J., Spirito, A., Little, T. D., & Grapentine, W. L. (2000). Peer functioning, family dysfunction, and psychological symptoms in a risk factor model for adolescent inpatients' suicidal ideation severity. *Journal of Clinical Child Psychology, 29*(3), 392–405.

Prinstein, M. J., Nock, M. K., Spirito, A., & Grapentine, W. L. (2001). Multimethod assessment of suicidality in adolescent psychiatric inpatients: Preliminary results. *Journal of the American Academy of Child and Adolescent Psychiatry, 40*(9), 1053–1061.

Rachlin, S. (1984). Double jeopardy: Suicide and malpractice. *General Hospital Psychiatry, 6*, 302–307.

Ramsay, J. R., & Newman, C. F. (2005). After the attempt: Maintaining the therapeutic alliance following a patient's suicide attempt. *Suicide and Life-Threatening Behavior, 35*(4), 413–424.

Reinecke, M. A., DuBois, D. L., & Schultz, T. M. (2001). Social problem solving, mood, and suicidality among inpatient adolescents. *Cognitive Therapy and Research, 25*(6), 743–756.

Reinert, D. F., & Allen, J. P. (2007). The Alcohol Use Disorders Identification Test: An update of research findings. *Alcoholism: Clinical and Experimental Research, 31*(2), 185–199.

Remafedi, G., French, S., Story, M., Resnick, M. D., & Blum, R. (1998). The relationship between suicide risk and sexual orientation: Results of a population-based study. *American Journal of Public Health, 88*(1), 57–60.

Resnick, M. D., Bearman, P. S., Blum, R. W., Bauman, K. E., Harris, K. M., Jones, J., et al. (1997). Protecting adolescents from harm: Findings from the National Longitudinal Study on Adolescent Health. *Journal of the American Medical Association, 278*(10), 823–832.

Reynolds, W. M. (1987). *Suicidal Ideation Questionnaire—Junior.* Odessa, FL: Psychological Assessment Resources.

Reynolds, W. M. (1988). *Suicidal Ideation Questionnaire: Professional manual.* Odessa, FL: Psychological Assessment Resources.

Reynolds, W. M. (2008). Reynolds Adolescent Depression Scale-2nd Edition: Short Form (RADS-2:SF). Lutz, FL: Psychological Assessment Resources, Inc.

Rhodes, K. V., Lauderdale, D. S., Stocking, C. B., Howes, D. S., Roizen, M. F., & Levinson, W. (2001). Better health while you wait: A controlled trial of a computer-based intervention for screening and health promotion in the emergency department. *Annals of Emergency Medicine, 37*(3), 284–291.

Roane, B. M., & Taylor, D. J. (2008). Adolescent insomnia as a risk factor for early adult depression and substance abuse. *Sleep: Journal of Sleep and Sleep Disorders Research, 31*(10), 1351–1356.

Roland, E. (2002). Bullying, depressive symptoms and suicidal thoughts. *Educational Research, 44*(1), 55–67.

Rooney, M. T., Fristad, M. A., Weller, E. B., & Weller, R. A. (1999). *Administration manual for the ChIPS.* Washington, DC: American Psychiatric Association.

Rotheram-Borus, M. J., & Bradley, J. (1991). Triage model for suicidal runaways. *American Journal of Orthopsychiatry, 61*(1), 122–127.

Rotheram-Borus, M. J., Piacentini, J., Cantwell, C., Belin, T. R., & Song, J. (2000). The 18-month impact of an emergency room intervention for adolescent female suicide attempters. *Journal of Consulting and Clinical Psychology, 68*(6), 1081–1093.

Rubenstein, J. L., Halton, A., Kasten, L., Rubin, C., & Stechler, G. (1998). Suicidal behavior in adolescents: Stress and protection in different family contexts. *American Journal of Orthopsychiatry, 68*(2), 274–284.

Rubenstein, J. L., Heeren, T., Housman, D., Rubin, C., & Stechler, G. (1989). Suicidal behavior in "normal" adolescents: Risk and protective factors. *American Journal of Orthopsychiatry, 59*(1), 59–71.

Rudd, M. D., Berman, A. L., Joiner, T. E., Jr., Nock, M. K., Silverman, M. M., Mandrusiak, M., et al. (2006). Warning signs for suicide: Theory, research, and clinical applications. *Suicide and Life-Threatening Behavior, 36*(3), 255–262.

Rudd, M. D., Joiner, T., & Rajab, M. H. (2001). *Treating suicidal behavior: An effective, time-limited approach.* New York: Guilford Press.

Rudd, M. D., Mandrusiak, M., & Joiner, T. E., Jr. (2006). The case against no-suicide contracts: The commitment to treatment statement as a practice alternative. *Journal of Clinical Psychology, 62*(2), 243–251.

Rudd, M. D., Rajab, M. H., Orman, D. T., Stulman, D. A., Joiner, T. E., Jr., & Dixon, W. (1996). Effectiveness of an outpatient intervention targeting suicidal young adults: Preliminary results. *Journal of Consulting and Clinical Psychology, 64*(1), 179–190.

Ruskin, R., Sakinofsky, I., Bagby, R. M., Dickens, S., & Sousa, G. (2004). Impact of patient suicide on psychiatrists and psychiatric trainees. *Academic Psychiatry, 28*(2), 104–110.

Russell, S. T., & Joyner, K. (2001). Adolescent sexual orientation and suicide risk: Evidence from a national study. *American Journal of Public Health, 91*(8), 1276–1281.

Safer, D. J. (1997). Self-reported suicide attempts by adolescents. *Annals of Clinical Psychiatry, 9*(4), 263–269.

Salzinger, S., Ng-Mak, D. S., Rosario, M., & Feldman, R. S. (2007). Adolescent suicidal behavior: Associations with preadolescent physical abuse and selected risk and protective factors. *Journal of the American Academy of Child and Adolescent Psychiatry, 46*(7), 859–866.

Sanci, L., Lewis, D., & Patton, G. (2010). Detecting emotional disorder in young people in primary care. *Current Opinion in Psychiatry, 23*(4), 318–323.

Sanford, M., Boyle, M., McCleary, L., Miller, J., Steele, M., Duku, E., et al. (2006). A pilot study of adjunctive family psychoeducation in adolescent major depression: Feasibility and treatment effect. *Journal of the American Academy of Child and Adolescent Psychiatry, 45*(4), 386–395.

Scherff, A. R., Eckert, T. L., & Miller, D. N. (2005). Youth suicide prevention: A survey of public school superintendents' acceptability of school-based programs. *Suicide and Life-Threatening Behavior, 35*(2), 154–169.

Scolte, R. H. J., van Lieshout, C. F. M., & van Aken, M. A. G. (2001). Perceived relational support in adolescence: Dimension, configurations, and adolescent adjustment. *Journal of Research on Adolescence, 11*(1), 71–94.

Scott, M. A., Wilcox, H. C., Schonfeld, S., Davies, M., Hicks, R. C., Tuner, J. B., et al. (2008). School-based screening to identify students not already known to school professionals: The Columbia Suicide Screen. *American Journal of Public Health, 99*, 1–6.

Shaffer, D. (1996). Predictive validity of the Suicide Probability Scale among adolescents in group home treatment: Discussion. *Journal of the American Academy of Child and Adolescent Psychiatry, 35*(2), 172–174.

Shaffer, D., Fisher, P., & Lucas, C. (2004). The Diagnostic Interview

Schedule for Children (DISC). In M. J. Hilsenroth & D. L. Segal (Eds.), *Comprehensive handbook of psychological assessment, Vol. 2: Personality assessment* (pp. 256–270). Hoboken, NJ: Wiley.

Shaffer, D., Gould, M. S., Fisher, P., & Trautman, P. (1996). Psychiatric diagnosis in child and adolescent suicide. *Archives of General Psychiatry, 53*(4), 339–348.

Shaffer, D., & Pfeffer, C. R. (2001). Practice parameter for the assessment and treatment of children and adolescents with suicidal behavior. *Journal of the American Academy of Child and Adolescent Psychiatry, 40*(Suppl. 7), 24S–51S.

Shaffer, D., Scott, M., Wilcox, H., Maslow, C., Hicks, R., Lucas, C. P., et al. (2004). The Columbia Suicide Screen: Validity and reliability of a screen for youth suicide and depression. *Journal of the American Academy of Child and Adolescent Psychiatry, 43*(1), 71–79.

Shafii, M., Carrigan, S., Whittinghill, J. R., & Derrick, A. (1985). Psychological autopsy of completed suicide in children and adolescents. *American Journal of Psychiatry, 142*(9), 1061–1064.

Shafii, M., Steltz-Lenarsky, J., Derrick, A. M., & Beckner, C. (1988). Comorbidity of mental disorders in the postmortem diagnosis of completed suicide in children and adolescents. *Journal of Affective Disorders, 15*(3), 227–233.

Shea, S. C. (1998a). The chronological assessment of suicide events: A practical interviewing strategy for the elicitation of suicidal ideation. *Journal of Clinical Psychiatry, 59*(Suppl. 20), 58–72.

Shea, S. C. (1998b). *Psychiatric interviewing: The art of understanding a practical guide for psychiatrists, psychologists, counselors, social workers, nurses, and other mental health professionals* (2nd ed.). Philadelphia: Saunders.

Shea, S. C. (2002). *The practical art of suicide assessment: A guide for mental health professionals and substance abuse counselors.* Hoboken, NJ: Wiley.

Sigfusdottir, I. D., Asgeirsdottir, B. B., Gudjonsson, G. H., & Sigurdsson, J. F. (2008). A model of sexual abuse's effects on suicidal behavior and delinquency: The role of emotions as mediating factors. *Journal of Youth and Adolescence, 37*(6), 699–712.

Silverman, M. M., Berman, A. L., Sanddal, N. D., O'Carroll, P. W., & Joiner, T. E. (2007). Rebuilding the tower of Babel: A revised nomenclature for the study of suicide and suicidal behaviors. Part 2: Suicide-related ideations, communications, and behaviors. *Suicide and Life-Threatening Behavior, 37*(3), 264–277.

Simon, R. I. (2001). *Concise guide to psychiatry and law for clinicians* (3rd ed.). Washington, DC: American Psychiatric Publishing.

Simon, R. I. (2002). Suicide risk assessment: What is the standard of care? *Journal of the American Academy of Psychiatry and the Law, 30*(3), 340–344.

Simon, R. I., & Shuman, D. W. (2009). Therapeutic risk management of clinical–legal dilemmas: Should it be a core competency? *Journal of the American Academy of Psychiatry and the Law, 37*(2), 155–161.

Stanley, B., & Brown, G. K. (2008). *Safety plan treatment manual to reduce suicide risk: Veteran's version.* Washington, DC: United States Department of Veteran's Affairs.

Stanley, B., & Brown, G. K. (2012). Safety planning intervention: A brief intervention to mitigate suicide risk. *Cognitive and Behavioral Practice, 19*(2), 256–264.

Stanley, B., Brown, G., Brent, D. A., Wells, K., Poling, K., Curry, J., et al. (2009). Cognitive-behavioral therapy for suicide prevention (CBT-SP): Treatment model, feasibility, and acceptability. *Journal of the American Academy of Child and Adolescent Psychiatry, 48*(10), 1005–1013.

Steer, R. A., Kumar, G., & Beck, A. T. (1993a). Hopelessness in adolescent psychiatric inpatients. *Psychological Reports, 72*(2), 559–-564.

Steer, R. A., Kumar, G., & Beck, A. T. (1993b). Self-reported suicidal ideation in adolescent psychiatric inpatients. *Journal of Consulting and Clinical Psychology, 61*(6), 1096–1099.

Strober, M., Schmidt-Lackner, S., Freeman, R., & Bower, S. (1995). Recovery and relapse in adolescents with bipolar affective illness: A five-year naturalistic, prospective follow-up. *Journal of the American Academy of Child & Adolescent Psychiatry, 34*(6), 724–731.

Suicide Prevention Resource Center. (2002). *National Violent Injury Statistics System fact sheet.* Retrieved February 25, 2011, from *www.sprc.org/library/YouthSuicideFactSheet.pdf.*

Suicide Prevention Resource Center. (2008). *Assessing and managing suicide risk: Core competencies for mental health professionals.* Newton, MA: Education Development Center.

Suicide Prevention Resource Center. (2012). *Recommendations for School-Based Suicide Prevention Screening.* Retrieved May 17th, 2012, from *www.sprc.org/sites/sprc.org/files/bpr/ScreeningRecommendations.pdf.*

TeenScreen Primary Care. (2012). *TeenScreen Primary Care: Guide to*

Coding and Payment. Retrieved May 23, 2012, from *www.teenscreen. org/images/stories/PDF/Guide-to-Coding-and-Payment-1-5-12.pdf.*

Thompson, E. A., Eggert, L. L., & Herting, J. R. (2000). Mediating effects of an indicated prevention program for reducing youth depression and suicide risk behaviors. *Suicide and Life-Threatening Behavior, 30*(3), 252–271.

Thompson, E. A., Eggert, L. L., Randell, B. P., & Pike, K. C. (2001). Evaluation of indicated suicide risk prevention approaches for potential high school dropouts. *American Journal of Public Health, 91*(5), 742–752.

Toros, F., Bilgin, N. G., Sasmaz, T., Bugdayci, R., & Camdeviren, H. (2004). Suicide attempts and risk factors among children and adolescents. *Yonsei Medical Journal, 45*(3), 367–374.

Tourangeau, R., & Yan, T. (2007). Sensitive questions in surveys. *Psychological Bulletin, 133*(5), 859–883.

Turner, C. F., Ku, L., Rogers, S. M., Lindberg, L. D., Pleck, J. H., & Sonenstein, F. L. (1998). Adolescent sexual behavior, drug use, and violence: Increased reporting with computer survey technology. *Science, 280*(5365), 867–873.

Tylee, A., Haller, D. M., Graham, T., Churchill, R., & Sanci, L. A. (2007). Youth-friendly primary-care services: How are we doing and what more needs to be done? *The Lancet, 369*(9572), 1565–1573.

U.S. Department of Health and Human Services. (2001). *National strategy for suicide prevention: Goals and objectives for action.* Rockville, MD: Public Health Service.

U.S. Public Health Service. (1999). *The Surgeon General's call to action to prevent suicide (1-23).* Washington, DC: Author.

Vandecreek, L., Knapp, S., & Herzog, C. (1987). Malpractice risks in the treatment of dangerous patients. *Psychotherapy, 24*(2), 145–153.

Velting, D. M., Shaffer, D., Gould, M. S., Garfinkel, R., Fisher, P., & Davies, M. (1998). Parent–victim agreement in adolescent suicide research. *Journal of the American Academy of Child and Adolescent Psychiatry, 37*(11), 1161–1166.

Vitaly Tarasoff et al. v. The Regents of the University of California et al., 551 P. 2d 334 (1976).

Wagner, B. M., Cole, R. E., & Schwartzman, P. (1996). Comorbidity of symptoms among junior and senior high school suicide attempters. *Suicide and Life-Threatening Behavior, 26*(3), 300–307.

Weist, M., Rubin, M., Moore, E., Adelsheim, S., & Wrobel, G. (2007).

Mental health screening in schools. *Journal of School Health, 77*(2), 53–58.

Welner, A., Welner, Z., & Fishman, R. (1979). Psychiatric adolescent inpatients: Eight- to ten-year follow-up. *Archives of General Psychiatry, 36*(6), 698–700.

Whetstone, L. M., Morrissey, S. L., & Cummings, D. M. (2007). Children at risk: The association between perceived weight status and suicidal thoughts and attempts in middle school youth. *Journal of School Health, 77*(2), 59.

Wilcox, H. C., Storr, C. L., & Breslau, N. (2009). Posttraumatic stress disorder and suicide attempts in a community sample of urban American young adults. *Archives of General Psychiatry, 66*(3), 305–311.

Wilkinson, P., Kelvin, R., Roberts, C., Dubicka, B., & Goodyer, I. (2011). Clinical and psychosocial predictors of suicide attempts and nonsuicidal self-injury in the Adolescent Depression Antidepressants and Psychotherapy Trial (ADAPT). *The American Journal of Psychiatry, 168*(5), 495–501.

Wills, T. A., & Cleary, S. D. (1996). How are social support effects mediated?: A test with parental support and adolescent substance use. *Journal of Personality and Social Psychology, 71*(5), 937–952.

Wilson, K. M., & Klein, J. D. (2000). Adolescents who use the emergency department as their usual source of care. *Archives of Pediatrics and Adolescent Medicine, 154*(4), 361–365.

Wintersteen, M. B. (2010). Standardized screening for suicidal adolescents in primary care. *Pediatrics, 125*(5), 938–944.

Wintersteen, M. B., Diamond, G., & Fein, J. (2007). Screening for suicide risk in the pediatric emergency and acute care setting. *Current Opinion in Pediatrics, 19*(4), 398–404.

Wunderlich, U., Bronisch, T., & Wittchen, H. U. (1998). Comorbidity patterns in adolescents and young adults with suicide attempts. *European Archives of Psychiatry and Clinical Neuroscience, 248*(2), 87–95.

Zenere, F. J., & Lazarus, P. J. (2009). The sustained reduction of youth suicidal behavior in a urban, multicultural school district. *School Psychology Review, 38*(2), 189–199.

Index

Page numbers in italics indicate tables or figures.

DU